Between the Regular and the Particular
in Speech and Language

Susanne Fuchs
Philip Hoole
Christine Mooshammer
Marzena Żygis
(eds.)

Between the Regular and the Particular in Speech and Language

PETER LANG
Frankfurt am Main · Berlin · Bern · Bruxelles · New York · Oxford · Wien

Bibliographic Information published by the Deutsche Nationalbibliothek
The Deutsche Nationalbibliothek lists this publication in the Deutsche Nationalbibliografie; detailed bibliographic data is available in the internet at http://dnb.d-nb.de.

Cover Design:
Olaf Glöckler, Atelier Platen, Friedberg

Cover Illustration:
Sandra Hashiguchi Pape, Costa Nova

ISBN 978-3-631-58686-0

www.peterlang.de

Contents

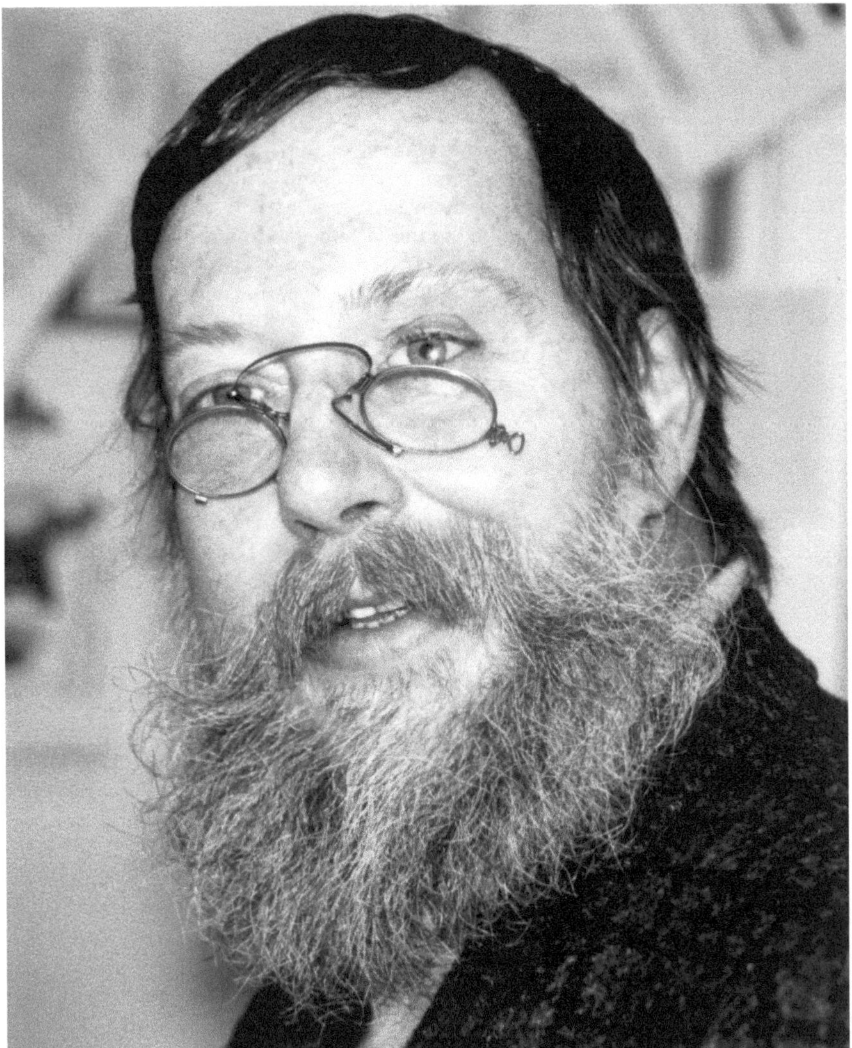

Figure 1. Bernd Pompino-Marschall (foto: Mariam Hartinger).

Editor's note: While casting around for material to illustrate the theme of the present volume we came across this illustration in the Proceedings of the 5th Speech Production Seminar. The editors of that volume attributed it to an artist of the late 20th century Pompino school. Despite considerable efforts we have been unable to pin it down more closely than that. The tempting assumption that the top part of the figure represents a self-portrait proved on the basis of internal evidence to be untenable. However this may be, the picture is apposite in several respects. Uncovering regularities in speech is an effortful process of chipping away at the raw material from different angles that, on the other hand, can never afford to ignore the particularities given by individual speaker anatomy (to name just one of many sources of variation in the speech chain). Probably all the contributions included in this volume give eloquent testimony to the tension between the regular and the particular in the analysis of speech. In so doing they highlight one respect in which the illustration is probably overly optimistic: It seems unlikely that knowledge about speech is likely to be set in stone for the foreseeable future.

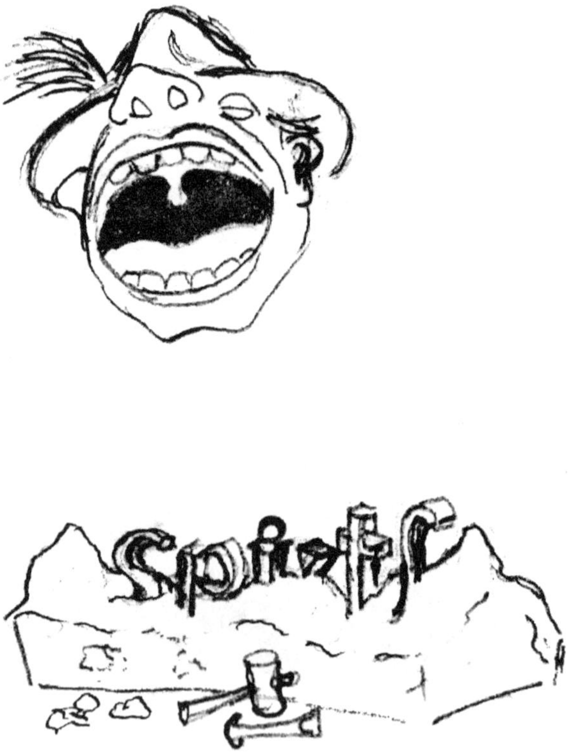

Laudationes

Dear Bernd, when we first met 18 years ago in the early summer of 1992 no one could have guessed that you would be moving from your Bavarian roots in Munich to make a permanent home in Berlin. In 1992 Berlin was marked by the massive changes brought about by the events of 1989 and was still in the process of linking up again its long separated eastern and western halves. Berlin's universities (Humboldt, Freie, Technische) were being radically reorganized and the former Akademie der Wissenschaften of the GDR was being wound up.

But the Akademie had one particular pearl, namely the Zentralinstitut für Sprachwissenschaften, with its excellent scientists and pre-eminent work. Small though it was, this major feature on the linguistic landscape was recommended by the Wissenschaftsrat for further support, and was destined to play an important role in the development of phonetics and phonology first in Berlin, but then in the whole of Germany. From January 1992 this provided the foundation for a new phase in the work of these disciplines. But there was a small problem! Back in the 1960s the subject of phonetics had been dropped at the Akademie der Wissenschaften. For more than 20 years phonetics had slumbered. There was no lab, not even a microphone, to say nothing of equipment for experimental phonetics such as articulograph, EPG, laryngograph, or transducer for intraoral air-pressure. The most expensive and sophisticated equipment amounted to a well-sharpened pencil! The installation of the first computers and internet connections was scheduled for 1992 ... The decision was taken to reanimate phonetics, and phonology along with it. Under the direction of Ewald Lang, a member of the Akademie of many years standing, the foundations for a modern phonetics lab and a phonetics/phonology research group were to be laid. And you, Bernd, at that time a young assistant of Prof. Tillmann at Munich University, successfully applied for the position of director of this new group, that was installed in 1992 as part of the research centre Allgemeine Sprachwissenschaft, Typologie und Universalienforschung under the aegis of the Max-Planck-Gesellschaft.

So began for me, an acoustics and electronics engineer, our many years of friendly and successful cooperation in establishing the phonetics lab.

Based in Jägerstraße in Berlin-Mitte you succeeded in a very short space of time in building up one of the main pillars of the research centre Allgemeine Sprachwissenschaft. As the lab's full-time director you continued for many years to ensure its further development, and still managed to find the time to supervise numerous significant new research projects in phonetics. In addition to all this hard work I also remember more curious occasions where your phonetic expertise sparked the interest of the mass-media, for example when your phonetic report as an expert witness saved the reputation of Bayern Munich goalkeeper Oliver Kahn when he was being hounded by reporters with allegations of racist abuse. Or the nurse from Neukölln (with a habit of dressing up as Till Eulenspiegel) who was fired from the hospital for allegedly making off with morphine from the drug trolley, but where the only grounds for suspicion came from her rough, rebellious tone of voice.
In the meantime we had mutated to the newly founded Zentrum für Allgemeine Sprachwissenschaft (ZAS) within the three Geisteswissenschaftliche Zentren and, supported by the Bundesland Berlin and the German Research Council, had acquired an international reputation.
Some years later the chair in phonetics at the Humboldt-University was advertised. I have many painful recollections of the difficulties you went through and the obstacles that had to be overcome before at last the professorship was yours.
Since then you have been busier than ever in your double position as professor and principal investigator at ZAS, and have had a major influence on the development of phonetics in Germany. Probably you alone can know just how many masters and doctoral candidates took their first scientific steps under your guidance. I gave up counting them, but have many vivid memories of them: the air-beds and late nights in the lab as the final touches were put to the theses, accompanied often by tears of joy and now and then by tears of worry.
Finally, I cannot forget to mention your dear wife Karin who followed you all the way from Munich those 18 years ago to your new home in Turmstrasse in Moabit.
I thank you for our collegial, friendly and successful collaboration over all those years of FAS, ZAS and HU.

Your engineer Jörg Dreyer

"Bernd Pompino-Marschall" For many years, this name was for me first and foremost the name of the author of a widely cited experimental study about perceptual centers (P-centers), published in 1989 in the Journal of Phonetics. Bernd's main contribution was twofold: he showed that the perception of momentary tempo was linked to the mean distance between two successive syllabic P-centers, and he proposed an algorithm to compute the location of the P-centers from a number of spectral events. This paper was thus destinated to become a reference for anyone wanting to work on the perception of timing in speech.
Hence, as I spoke to him the first time, during his visit to Grenoble in 1988, I did so with lots of respect and admiration. Beside his scientific skills, I was impressed by his manner of speaking German, slowly, precisely, with eloquence, with a rich vocabulary, and also with a kind of old-fashion speaking style. With his long beard and his glasses that looked like monocle, Bernd reminded me of the pictures of the famous scientists of the beginning of the 20th century, which decorate the walls of many prestigious German universities.
Since then we have met several times, we worked together, and I discovered the man, hearty, cultivated, generous, thoughtful, loving life and people. I especially remember a wonderful evening with him and his wife Karin in a typical German restaurant in Munich with lots of beer and laughter, or a dinner in a restaurant of the, to me, impressive Alexanderplatz, just after he left Munich to become the head of the Phonetic Group at the ZAS, the Center for General Linguistics, in Berlin. Spending an evening with Bernd is always a big pleasure. He makes everyone feel good, he has humor and he always has interesting stories to tell, among other things, about Germany, German culture and German phonetics.
I am very grateful to Bernd that he proposed to me in 1999 to be an external collaborator on his DFG Grant about Speech Production and Perception. It gave me the opportunity to work with a number of (at this time) young and (still now) enthusiastic scientists and wonderful persons: Tine Mooshammer, Susanne Fuchs, Christian Geng, Sabine Koppetsch, Daniel Pape, and Jörg Dreyer. I had a wonderful time with these colleagues. I learned a lot, I established very close collaborations and we launched all together a number of research projects that are still going on now. I spent a number weeks in the old building of the ZAS in

the Jägerstrasse and I could observe how Bernd managed his lab, and his collaborators. I think that he belongs to the rare kind of directors and professors who are thoughtful without being paternalist, supportive without being directive, wise without being bossy. He has created for these scientists the conditions for them to blossom scientifically, and all of them did him proud. Beside his other contributions to phonetics, the creation and the development of this phonetics lab, is certainly a major contribution of Bernd Pompino-Marschall to science, and to the durability of phonetic research in Germany.

Pascal Perrier, Grenoble

Phonological Length of Number Marking Morphemes in the Framework of Typological Markedness

JANA BRUNNER*

Abstract: The study tests the hypothesis that morphemes marking the typologically less marked member of the conceptual category of number should have a phonological length that is less than or equal to that of morphemes marking a typologically more marked member of the same category. The hypothesis is tested for morphemes marking number in nouns, verbs, adjectives and pronouns. The cross-linguistic quantitative count includes 42 languages, 17 of them exhibiting a singular-plural-dual contrast, the others having a singular-plural contrast only. In order to measure phonological length the phonemes making up a morpheme are counted. The hypothesis is verified: Apart from rare exceptions, singular markers have for all the four parts of speech a length that is less than or equal to that of the corresponding plural markers. In languages with dual markers these are longer than or equally long as the corresponding plural and singular markers.

1 Introduction

The concept of markedness was first developed in the Prague School of linguistic theory (Trubetzkoy, 1931, 1969; Jakobson, 1932, 1939) where it described a language internal property of category values. A marked and an unmarked member of a category, for example the category of number, are in *privative opposition*: one category value (e.g. singular for the category of number) is characterized by the absence, the other by the presence of a mark (e.g. plural). When the concept of markedness was taken over into typology by Greenberg in 1966 this involved important changes. Typological markedness is now no longer a property

* For Bernd, something completely unrelated to palates. With many thanks for the support during my thesis work, for interesting discussions, for being there without being pushy, for giving room to develop independence, for an atmosphere of trust.

of a language specific category but a universal property of a conceptual category, and it is not necessarily binary (Croft, 1996, p.17). Typological markedness would thus not claim that, within the category of number, the singular is unmarked in one or the other language, but that crosslinguistically the value singular is the unmarked value of the conceptual category of number, plural is more marked and other values such as dual are even more marked.

Croft (2003, ch.4) sets up a number of *criteria of* (typological) *markedness*, i.e. *structural coding*, *behavioral potential* and *text frequency*. According to the first criterion, the typologically marked value of a grammatical category will be expressed by at least as many morphemes as the typologically unmarked value of that category (Croft, 2003, p.92). As a consequence of that, for the category of number, one logically possible configuration, i.e. overtly marked singular and zero-coded plural, is excluded by the markedness criterion of structural coding. And cross-linguistic comparison shows that this type is indeed very rare (Croft, 2003, p.89). The second criterion of markedness, *behavioral potential* describes the "grammatical versatility" (Croft, 2003, p.95) of values of a category. Behavioral potential can manifest itself in the number of morphological categorical distinctions that a particular category value possesses: The typologically unmarked value of a category will have at least as many formal distinctions in a given inflectional paradigm as the marked value (Croft, 2003, p.97). To give an example from English, there is a gender distinction in singular personal pronouns but not in plural personal pronouns, suggesting that the singular is less marked.

Text frequency presents the third criterion and at the same time the explanatory variable of typological markedness. The tokens of the unmarked value of a category occur at least as frequently as the tokens of the marked value (Croft, 2003, p.110). Greenberg (1966, p.32, 37) demonstrates the greater frequency of the singular as compared to (the dual and) the plural by a quantitative count of nouns and verbs in written speech. Following this analysis the singular is in all languages the most frequently occurring value of the category. In Sanskrit, which has a dual marker, this latter marker occurs least frequently.

According to Croft (2003, ch.4), the criteria of markedness are not independent from each other, they are the result of the competing motivations of *economy* and *iconicity*. Economy suggests that expressions should be minimized where possible, whereas iconicity proposes that the structure of language should reflect the structure of human experience. This means that there should be a one-to-one mapping of conceptual values onto form (i.e. one marker for each conceptual value). Again applied to the category of number this means that overt marking for both singular and plural is maximally iconically motivated but minimally economically motivated since it reflects the structure of experience but demands a high degree of articulatory effort. On the other hand, the other three types (zero marking for one or both category values) are economically motivated but not iconically. Zero marking for both singular and plural demands a low degree of articulatory effort (therefore this type is economic); however, there are no markers in language which reflect the two category values which are experienced in the world (therefore this type is not iconic). The two asymmetric types, zero-marking for one member of the category and overt marking for the other member are not iconic either, but moderately economic. This, however, does not explain why one asymmetric type (overt marking of singular, zero marking of plural) is so rare and the other one so frequent. Looking at the frequency of the category values, however, can explain this pattern: because the singular is much more frequent than the plural it is actually highly uneconomic to use overt marking for the singular and zero marking for the plural; it is much more economic to do it the other way round. The difference in frequency thus explains the difference in structural coding.

Other approaches have questioned the role of iconicity in the formation of linguistic structure (Haspelmath, 2008a), and even claimed that the concept of typological markedness is superfluous (Haspelmath, 2006). Haspelmath (2006) claims that the observed phenomena can be explained entirely by language external factors, particularly by frequency of use. The differences in structural coding exist because, for reasons of economy, speakers will either shorten frequent items, or they will use the base form to denote a frequent item and add a further marker for the less frequent form (Haspelmath, 2006, p.48). The differences in singular and plural marking thus come about because speakers either shorten the more frequent form or attach a marker to the less frequent form. Haspelmath claims that the concept of typological markedness is not needed in order to explain these data.

Frequency of use alone can, according to Haspelmath, also explain what has been called "markedness reversal" in the literature on typological markedness; i.e. cases in which the category value which is usually less marked (e.g. singular) occurs less often than the more marked alternative. As an example, Haspelmath (2008b, p.61) discusses singular/plural pairs such as *criterion-criteria*, where the plural is more frequent and therefore shorter than the singular.

Haspelmath (2008b, p.59) adds predictability as a factor shaping grammatical structure: If an item is frequent (as most singular forms are) it is usually predictable and thus receives less and less overt coding until it is finally zero coded. If items are rarer (as are plural or dual forms) they keep their overt coding because rarer forms are less predictable and therefore need overt coding.

Given the importance of frequency in shaping overt coding one could assume that a language arrives at the most frequently observed constellation (zero marking for singular and overt marking for plural) by either shortening the more frequent marker of two or more existing markers until it is finally lost for economic reasons. An alternative scenario would be that a plural marker comes into existence to distinguish between singular and plural (for reasons of iconicity or because of a lack of predictability).

Following from the assumption that the very frequent typologically less marked category markers are shortened and finally get lost over time, it has been hypothesized that structural coding would be sensitive to phonological length as well as morphological length: An overtly coded unmarked value of a category should not be phonologically longer than the overtly coded marked value (Dryer, cited in Croft, 2003: 115f). Morphologically longer means that plural forms consist of more morphemes than singular forms; phonologically longer means that they consist of more phonological material (e.g. segments).

Differences in morphological length can come about in the two ways discussed above, either by the creation of a morpheme for the more marked category (possibly due to iconic considerations) or by shortening a frequent morpheme until it is finally lost for reasons of economy. Differences in phonological length can only come about by shortening an existing marker due to economic reasons.

The aim of the present study is to test the hypothesis that typologically more marked members of the category of number are coded by markers which are at least as long as the markers of the typologically less marked members of the category. It will be investigated whether, for overt coding only, plural morphemes consist of at least as many segments as singular markers and whether dual markers consist of at least as many segments as plural and singular markers. This hypothesis will be tested on number markers on verbs, nouns, adjectives and pronouns in 42 languages from all parts of the world. In contrast to counts including morphological length the present analysis investigates the influence of economy on number marking morphemes separately from the influence of iconicity (which could lead to the creation of markers for one or the other category).

There are a number of earlier studies which have investigated phonological (and usually also morphological) length. Stolz et al. (2006) carried out a study on comitative and instrumental markers. For a sample of 217 languages with distinct markers for comitative and instrumental they found that comitative markers are longer (more segments and/or syllables) than instrumental markers in 62.7% of the cases and shorter in 27.2% of the cases (p.173f). If the comitative was longer than the instrumental the ratio was on average 1:2 for segments and syllables. If the comitative was shorter than the instrumental the ratio was about 1:1.7.

Stolz et al. (2007) did a similar study on lexical duals in 120 languages. They argue that the definite numeral denoting two elements (engl. *both*) is semantically more complex than the indefinite numeral (engl. *two*), since it not only quantifies the noun, as does the indefinite numeral, but also determines it. Following from that, the definite numeral should also be morphologically and phonologically more complex. They counted the number of morphemes, segments and syllables in indefinite numerals denoting two elements (engl. *two*) and definite numerals (engl. *both*). The analysis shows that in the overwhelming majority of cases the definite numeral consisted of more segments (76.3%), more syllables (77% of the cases) and more morphemes (60.8%, Stolz et al. (2007, p.171)).

Stolz et al. (2010) investigated the markedness relation between comitative/instrumental and abessives. Starting from an analysis of semantic complexity of these markers the hypothesis was set up that the abessive should be the marked category value and should therefore have at least as much structural coding as the comitative/instrumental. A count of morphological and phonological length on 212 morphemes in 74 languages (number of morphemes, syllables and segments) showed that the abessive is phonologically and morphologically at least as long as the comitative and instrumental markers. 80% of the abessive morphemes consisted of more segments than the corresponding comitative or instrumental morphemes, 85% had more syllables and 75% had more morphemes (Stolz et al., 2010, ch. 3.2.1).

2 Methods

2.1 Aim of the study

The aim of this cross-linguistic study is to find out whether typologically less marked members of the category of number are expressed by phonologically shorter or equally long markers than more marked members of the category; more specifically, whether the phonological length of singular markers is less than or equal to that of plural and dual markers and whether the length of plural markers is less than or equal to that of dual markers. Because trial and paucal are extremely rare in the languages of the world and it is consequently very hard to get a sample large enough for this analysis they will be ignored in the present study. Phonological length will be measured in two different ways: as the number of segments (phonemes) and number of syllables. The method is similar to earlier studies (Stolz et al., 2010), except that, in order to measure phonological length only, morphemes are not counted. The following data will be obtained:

- the percentages of markers of a member of the category of number that are longer, shorter or equally long as compared to markers marking other members of the category (syllables and segments),
- the absolute number of cases in which a marker marking one member of the category is longer, shorter or equally long as compared to markers marking other members of the category (syllables and segments),
- the average difference in phonemes and syllables for cases in which the morphemes are not equally long.

2.2 Language sample

The sample consists of number marking morphemes from 42 geographically distant languages which are not closely related, 17 of them showing a singular/plural/dual contrast and 25 a singular/plural contrast only. Sampling closely followed the method proposed by Dryer (1989, 1992): Only one language from a genus was taken and the languages were apportioned about equally to six large linguistic areas (Dryer, 1992, p.83). Languages were classified following Ruhlen (1991). Table 1 gives the language sample of the present study. The languages are preceded by their genus.

Table 1. Language sample

Africa	**Australia and New Guinea**
1 Semitic: Arabic	22 Gunwinyguan: Wardaman
2 Gur: Supyire	23 Mabuso: Amele
3 Southern West Atlantic: Kisi	24 Dani-Kwerba: Lower Grand Valley Dani
4 Nilotic: Turkana	25 Nor-Pondo: Yimas
5 Bantu: Tswana	26 Wapei-Palei: Olo
6 Central Khoisan: Nama	27 Pama-Nyungan: Guugu Yimidhirr
7 Biu-Mandara: Hdi'	28 Solomons: Lavukaleve
Eurasia	**North America**
8 Turkic: Karachay	29 Eskimo-Aleut: West Greenlandic
9 Ugric: Hungarian	30 Athapaskan-Eyak: Slave (Hare dialect)
10 Basque: Basque	31 Coast Salish: Upriver Halkomelem
11 Celtic: Breton	32 Algonquian: Blackfoot
12 Slavic: Russian	33 Muskogean: Koasati
13 Dravidian Proper: Malayalam	34 Aztecan: Classical Nahuatl
14 Munda: Santali	35 Mayan: Tzutujil
South-East Asia and Oceania	**South America**
15 Tibetic: Athpare	36 Mura: Wari
16 Oceanic: Tinrin	37 Peba-Yaguan: Yagua
17 Burmese-Lolo: Bisu	38 Arawan: Paumari
18 Central Malayo Polynesian: Kambera	39 Guaicuruan: Toba
19 Sulawesi Austronesian: Tukang Besi	40 Paya: Paya (Pech)
20 Aslian: Semelai	41 Araucanian: Mapudungun
21 Atayalic: Atayal	42 Waicari-Qinigua: Kadiwé

2.3 Choice of morphemes and determination of length differences

The term *morpheme* refers to bound morphemes as well as free morphemes. With regard to verbs, nouns and adjectives, only bound morphemes are considered in the present study. The verbal morphemes used in this study mark agreement with the subject or object, the nominal morphemes mark the number of the denoted element, the adjectival morphemes mark agreement with the noun modified by the adjective. Pronominal markers used in this study are all free morphemes. The bound morphemes sometimes called "pronouns" in the grammars which can be attached to verbs as person/number markers would be treated as verbal morphemes.
As stated in the introduction, number marking usually involves zero marking for at least one member of the category. Since the present study does not compare morphological but phonological length, however, only overt markers will be considered. Cases where there is a zero and an overtly marked form (e.g. English number marking on nouns) will not be considered. The reason for this is that when a value is coded by zero length, one cannot differentiate between morphological length and phonological length.
For languages with a singular-dual-plural contrast, if there is zero marking for one value of the category (usually the singular), but overt marking for the other two categories, the two overt markers will be compared and the zero marker will be ignored. An example is given for Arabic (Holes, 1995, p.134, example 1). Here the dual and plural are overtly marked and will be included in the analysis, but the singular is zero marked and will therefore be ignored.

1. SG: *mudi:r*
   DU(Nominative): *mudi:ra:ni*
   PL(Nominative): *mudi:ru:na*

Ideally, the morphemes used in this study should only mark number. However, for reasons of economy, those morphemes are very rare. Often, morphemes marking number mark at the same time person, tense or aspect on verbs, or case on nouns. There are only three languages in the sample with number markers only marking number: Tinrin, Bisu and

Wardaman. To give just one example, Wardaman has the dual markers *–guya* or *–wuya,* which only mark dual and can be affixed to either noun or verb, and the plural markers *–mulu* and *–bulu* (Merlan, 1994, p.90):

2. *ngayi-ga-n-guya*
   1INDU-take-PRES-DU
   'Let's you and I take it.'

3. *dan-mulu goyogba-mulu wurre-mulu yibiyi-wagbwun*
   this-PL orphan-PL-ABS child-PL-ABS father-lacking-ABS
   'These are orphans, [they have] no father.' [1]

In contrast to these languages, however, most languages have number markers which mark something else apart from number. If there are more of these morphemes available than are needed for the present study morphemes which mark the unmarked category members of other categories were preferred over morphemes marking a marked member (for example, indicative markers rather than subjunctive markers, markers of subject agreement rather than object agreement, active voice rather than passive). Tzutujil, for example, has nominal number markers which at the same time mark absolutive or ergative case and person (table 2).

Table 2. Number marking on Tzutujil nouns (Dayley, 1985, p.62)

CASE/PERSON	SINGULAR	PLURAL
ABSOLUTIVE		
1st	*in-*	*og-*
2nd	*at-*	*ix-*
ERGATIVE, PRECONSONANTAL		
1st	*nuu-*	*gaa-*
2nd	*aa-*	*ee-*
3rd	*ruu-*	*kee-*
ERGATIVE, PREVOCALIC		
1st	*w-*	*q-*
2nd	*aaw-*	*eew-*
3rd	*r-*	*k-*

Here the absolutive person markers are used rather than the ergative markers. Sometimes not a complete paradigm can be considered. In

Russian number marking on male nouns, there is zero marking in the nominative and accusative singular. Therefore, only the other cases were used (table 3).

Table 3. Declination of Russian masculine nouns (Morris et al., 1996, p.442)

	SINGULAR	PLURAL
Nominative	*stol* 'table'	*stol-y*
Genitive	*stol-a*	*stol-ov*
Dative	*stol-u*	*stol-am*
Accusative	*stol*	*stol-y*
Instrumental	*stol-om*	*stol-ami*
Prepositional	*stol-e*	*stol-ax*

Very often one finds more than one singular form for only one plural form. In the Turkana example (table 4) there are only two forms in the plural as opposed to three in the singular. This is because the singular has a greater behavioral potential (see introduction). In those cases all the singular forms are compared with the respective plural forms separately. In the Turkana example this means that the two feminine forms were compared with each other, the masculine singular form was compared with the masculine/neuter plural form and the neuter singular form with the masculine/neuter plural form. This of course applies not only to gender contrasts but also to all other cases in which the greater behavioral potential of a value of the category of number shows up.

Table 4. Number marking on countable nouns in Turkana (Dimmendaal, 1983, p.210)

	SINGULAR	PLURAL
Feminine	*a-*	*ŋa-*
Masculine	*e-*	*ŋi-*
Neuter	*i-*	*ŋi-*

As stated above, the category of number can have different numbers of members depending on the language. The singular always denotes one referent and the dual two. The value plural, however, can have different meanings in the different languages. It can determine more than one element, but in dual languages possibly only more than two. In Wardaman the plural which refers to more than one element is called *non-singular,* the plural which denotes more than two elements is called *plural* (table 5). Those differences are ignored here; *plural* as it is used here includes both meanings. The non-singular in the Wardaman example is treated as plural.

Table 5. Wardaman pronouns, base form (Merlan, 1994, p.122)

SINGULAR		DUAL		PLURAL		NONSINGULAR	
1	*ngayug-bi*	1IN	*yawung-guya-wi*	1IN	*ngarrug-bi*	1EX	*yurrug-bi*
2	*yinyang-bi*	2	*nurrug-(g)uya-wi*	2	*nurrug-bulu-wi*	2	*nurrug-bi*
3	*narnaj-bi*	3	*narnay-guya-wi*	3	*narnay-bulu-wi*		

Some languages mark one value of the category of number by an umlaut. In Olo, for example, one finds plural marking on nouns with affixes and umlaut (McGregor and McGregor, 1982, p.30):

4. *sengke* 'pig'
   songkou 'pigs'

Those cases are ignored since there is no clear boundary between stem and number marker and it is not possible to count differences in phonological length (Croft, 2003, p.94).

Inflectional paradigms often have cases of suppletion. Suppletion is a phenomenon which does not occur equally often in all areas of the world (Veselinova, 2005a,b). Ignoring suppletive forms completely could therefore have led to a bias in our corpus. However, similarly to the cases with umlaut marking, for bound morphemes it is often not possible to determine the boundary between stem and affix in suppletive forms. Therefore, cases with stem suppletion are not included in the sample. For pronominal markers, which are free morphemes, suppletive forms were included because the complete word was counted. For the same reason, number marking by inner modification and suprasegmentals was excluded.

Number can furthermore be marked by reduplication. One could say that in this case phonological material is added to the stem. However, what is added is not an independent morpheme (Croft, 2003, p.95) so its status is questionable. This led to the exclusion of these cases from the present count.

Sometimes the form of a morpheme which is added to a stem depends on the semantics of the word. Those systems can be very complex. In these cases the most frequent type(s) were chosen. To illustrate this, an example from Kisi is given (table 6).

Table 6. Number marking on Kisi nouns (Childs, 1995, p.148)

-ó	singular of all animates, some inanimates
-á	plural of animates
-léŋ	singular of inanimates
-láŋ	plural of inanimates
-é	singular of collective plants
-óŋ	plural of collective grains, etc.
-áŋ	liquids

Each Kisi noun belongs to one of seven classes which are defined semantically. Some classes are singular, some are plural, and some seem to be neither one nor the other. The first column in the following list gives the suffix of the nouns in the class, the second a semantic characterization. Some of these noun classes can be paired, so that a pair consists of a singular class denoting certain elements and a plural class denoting the same class of elements. Childs (1995) also gives the frequency of the respective pairings (table 7).

Table 7. Number marking on Kisi nouns (Childs, 1995, p.149)

SINGULAR	PLURAL	PERCENTAGES OF TOTAL PAIRING
-ó	*-láŋ*	43.4%
-ó	*-á*	27.3%
-é	*-óŋ*	15.3%
-léŋ	*-é*	4.3%
-léŋ	*-láŋ*	3.2%
-léŋ	*-áŋ*	3.1%
-ó	*-é*	3.0%
-léŋ	*-óŋ*	0.3%

As one can see, some pairings are very rare and are therefore ignored in the present study. Only the first, second and third pairing are included in the analysis since they occur most frequently. This method differs from Stolz et al. (2010)'s investigation of the markedness relation between comitative/instrumental and abessive. Their sample includes on the one hand languages with different markers for the first two categories but only one for the abessive, and on the other hand languages with only one marker for both comitative and instrumental. In the first case, Stolz et al. selected the shorter marker from the first two categories. Since, however, the aim of the present study was to investigate this very parameter, the length of the markers, it was decided to take all markers except for the very rare ones.

Following Haspelmath (2006, p.56), frequency can result in articulatory simplicity of the item. As a consequence, articulatorily difficult phonetic segments should occur more often in rarer morphemes than in frequent ones. So the articulatory difficulty of the segments should actually be taken into account in the present study. However, for practical reasons it was decided not to do so because it was impossible to set up a ranking of sounds as to their articulatory difficulty. Whereas most people will agree that certain classes of sounds (such as ejectives) are more complex than others, for the purposes of this study it would have been necessary to decide whether the difference in complexity between two given sounds is greater than the difference between two other given sounds, which is not easily possible. Articulatory complexity certainly influences shortening of the morphemes marking less marked category values, but the present study restricts itself to a discussion of phonological length.

The phonemes which make up a morpheme were counted. A singleton consonant was counted as one unit, as was a monophthong. Vowels with length markers, diphthongs and consonantal geminates were counted as two units. This partly follows Stolz et al. (2010, ch.3.2.1) who counted diphthongs as two elements. The reasoning behind this is that segment length plays a role in language change, so one can assume that it plays a role in the process which is under investigation here, namely, whether morphemes marking more marked members of a category are shortened more easily than less marked morphemes of the category.

2.4 Determining phonological length within a language

In most cases not all the parts of speech of a chosen language exhibit overt number marking by suitable morphemes. Therefore very often markers for one, two or three parts of speech only are considered. Moreover, sometimes only very few morphemes are chosen from one part of speech of one language, in other cases very many morphemes are taken because very many suitable morphemes could be found. In order to avoid a biasing of the data due to different numbers of morphemes for different parts of speech or languages phonological length is measured separately first for each language (or genus, since one language represents one genus), second for each area and only finally for all the areas together. The parts of speech are counted separately throughout the whole study.

An example for the count within a language and part of speech will be given. In Russian nominal inflection (masculine, inanimate nouns, see table 3) the nominative and accusative are zero-marked in the singular. Therefore, they are not considered any further. In each of the remaining pairs of morphemes the singular form is one phoneme shorter than the plural. In one case the singular is also one syllable shorter. Furthermore, the average difference in number of segments (or syllables) between the plural and singular forms is 1 and 1, respectively. The result of this count is summarized in table 8.

Table 8. Result for number marking on nouns in Russian. First column: relationship between two members of a category, second column: percentage of cases in which this relationship was found and – in parentheses – absolute number of cases. Third and fourth column: results for syllables.

	SEGMENTS		SYLLABLES	
	Percentage	Average difference	Percentage	Average difference
SG<PL	100% (4)	1	25% (1)	1
SG=PL	0% (0)		75% (3)	
SG>PL	0% (0)		0% (0)	

The first column in this table gives the relationship between two members of the category. The second and third columns refer to segments, the last two columns to syllables. The second and fourth column give the percentages of cases and – in parenthesis – the absolute number of cases. The third and fifth column show the average difference in the number of segments/syllables.

All the languages from the different genera are now grouped according to the linguistic areas they belong to (see the list of languages in table 1). For each part of speech the average percentages of morphemes are counted which are longer, shorter or equally long in one value as compared to the other(s). The numbers of cases are added and the average difference in length is counted. Finally, a mean over the six linguistic areas is calculated (percentages and numbers of average difference). The numbers of cases are added.

3 Results and discussion

Tables 9 to 12 show the results for each part of speech (verbs, nouns, adjectives, pronouns). In the overwhelming majority of cases the phonological length of the singular is less than or equal to the length of the plural or the dual, and the length of the plural is less than or equal to the one of the dual. The data thus support the hypothesis.

There are more interesting facts that can be seen from those figures which all show that markedness (and with it the explanatory variable frequency) strongly influences phonological length. The first observation concerns the average difference in length which is overall greater in cases that prove the hypothesis right than in cases that prove it wrong. To give an example, for verbs the average difference for cases in which the length of the singular is less than or equal to that of the plural (predicted case) is 1.3 segments whereas in the unpredicted case (singular longer than plural) it is only 1.0 (table 9). The only exception to that is the average difference in syllables for verbs which is 1.0 for both the predicted and the unpredicted case (table 9). Relating this observation to frequency one can say that if a more frequent form is longer than a less frequent form (unpredicted case) the difference in length is usually smaller than if a less frequent form is longer than a more frequent form (predicted case). The reason for that could again be that more frequent forms are shortened more easily than less frequent forms. This is consistent with Stolz et al. (2006, p.174); they showed that if the less marked instrumental is shorter, it is half as long as the more marked comitative, but if the comitative is shorter, the difference between instrumental and comitative is smaller.

The average difference between singular and dual is greater than the av-

Table 9. Result for verbs. Columns as in table 8.

	SEGMENTS Percentage	Average difference	SYLLABLES Percentage	Average difference
SG<PL	41% (48)	1.3	18% (21)	1
SG=PL	54% (61)		81% (91)	
SG>PL	5% (4)	1	1% (1)	1
SG<DU	59% (19)	1.9	36% (14)	1
SG=DU	41% (14)		64% (19)	
SG>DU	0% (0)		0% (0)	
PL<DU	45% (16)	1.36	10% (8)	1.06
PL=DU	49% (25)		90% (35)	
PL>DU	6% (2)	1	0% (0)	

Table 10. As table 9 but for nouns.

	SEGMENTS Percentage	Average difference	SYLLABLES Percentage	Average difference
SG<PL	57% (42)	1.62	35% (26)	1.11
SG=PL	36% (26)		59% (43)	
SG>PL	7% (8)	1.57	6% (7)	1
SG<DU	88% (12)	1.8	75% (12)	1.22
SG=DU	12% (1)		25% (1)	
SG>DU	0% (0)		0% (0)	
PL<DU	59% (7)	1.2	27% (7)	1.0
PL=DU	41% (13)		73% (13)	
PL>DU	0% (0)		0% (0)	

erage differences between singular and plural or plural and dual: The mean value of the averages for singular<dual is 1.93 across parts of speech (segments) and 1.12 (syllables). The numbers for singular<plural (1.48/1.04) and plural<dual (1.51/1.11) are lower. The reason for that could be that there is a greater difference in frequency between singular and dual than between singular vs. plural and dual vs. plural.

Looking a little closer at the cases that run counter to the hypothesis one can find even more evidence for the singular<plural<dual hierarchy in typological markedness. Following from the greater inequalities in frequency between singular and dual than between singular vs. plural and dual vs. plural, there should be fewer unpredicted cases in the singular

vs. dual comparison than in the singular vs. plural and plural vs. dual comparisons.

Table 11. As table 9 but for adjectives.

	SEGMENTS Percentage	Average difference	SYLLABLES Percentage	Average difference
SG<PL	27% (9)	1.25	27% (7)	1
SG=PL	68% (17)		62% (18)	
SG>PL	5% (2)	1	11% (3)	1
SG<DU	100% (6)	1.88	75% (4)	1
SG=DU	0% (0)		25% (2)	
SG>DU	0% (0)		0% (0)	
PL<DU	83% (6)	1.75	75% (5)	1.17
PL=DU	17% (2)		25% (3)	
PL>DU	0% (0)		0% (0)	

In fact this tendency can be seen. Whereas in up to 8% for segments and 11% for syllables (tables 12 and 11) the singular is longer than the plural and in up to 17% (table 12, segments, no cases for syllables) the plural is longer than the dual, there are only two cases (2%, table 12) in which the singular is longer than the dual (looking at segments, not looking at syllables).

Table 12. As table 9 but for pronouns.

	SEGMENTS Percentage	Average difference	SYLLABLES Percentage	Average difference
SG<PL	53% (67)	1.73	34% (45)	1.03
SG=PL	39% (49)		62% (75)	
SG>PL	8% (8)	1	4% (4)	1
SG<DU	75% (30)	2.13	74% (29)	1.27
SG=DU	23% (13)		26% (16)	
SG>DU	2% (2)	1	0% (0)	
PL<DU	51% (20)	1.2	25% (14)	1.21
PL=DU	32% (22)		75% (39)	
PL>DU	17% (11)	1.13	0% (0)	

From all these observations the following conclusion can be drawn.

There seems to be a connection between differences in the phonological length of the forms of two values and differences in markedness. If there is a great difference in markedness (like in the relation singular vs. dual) then there is a great difference in phonological length (average length and percentages of cases). If the difference in markedness is smaller (dual vs. plural and singular vs. plural) then the difference in phonological length is smaller.

Regarding the differences between segments and syllables, there is a tendency to have no difference in syllables but a difference in segments. In other words, typically the plural has more segments than the singular but not more syllables, and the same applies to the relation dual vs. plural. For the relation singular vs. dual the dual has typically both more syllables and more segments. Moreover, the average differences in segments are greater than the differences in syllables.

Looking at the parts of speech the following preferences can be discovered. Nouns and pronouns typically exhibit singular ≤ plural (depending on whether one looks at segments or syllables), singular < dual and plural ≤ dual, (tables 10 and 12). Verbs and adjectives support the hypothesis less than nouns and pronouns. Verbs have singular = plural, singular ≤ dual and plural = dual (table 9). For adjectives the relations are singular = plural, singular < dual and plural < dual (table 11). One could again try to find a reason for that by looking at frequency. Nouns should, following from this result, occur more often in the singular than for example verbs. However, according to the counts given in Greenberg (1966, p.32,37) the opposite seems to be the case. According to Greenberg, percentages for singular and plural forms in different parts of speech vary across languages, and for three out of four languages the percentages for singular forms of verbs are higher than the ones for nouns. For Latin, for example, Greenberg gives the following figures for singular: 91% of the verbs and 85.2% for nouns.

Pronouns have the highest percentage of cases contradicting the markedness hierarchy (SG>PL: 8/4%, SG>DU: 2/0%, PL>DU 17/0%). In some cases these results can be explained by the existence of several alternatives (inclusive and exclusive) in dual and/or plural. In Hdi' pronouns, for example, there are inclusive and exclusive forms in the plural but not in the dual. The exclusive plural form is longer than the dual form. An explanation for that could be that if there are two alternatives each of those has a lower frequency than a single form would have. So each form will be shortened less than it would have been if it was the only form.

4 Summary

The aim of the present study was to test the hypothesis that typologically more marked (and thus less frequent) markers of the category of number are phonologically longer than or equally long as markers of typlogically less marked (and thus less frequent) members of the category. The results of this study demonstrate that even when there is no difference in morphological length, there is a difference in phonological length between the typologically marked values and typologically unmarked values. Furthermore, the results are in agreement with an explanation of structural coding in terms of economy. There is a greater economic motivation to shorten the more frequent and less marked forms than to shorten the less frequent and more marked forms.

The count included 42 languages, each of them from a different genus. The languages/genera were divided into six large linguistic areas which were analyzed separately first before calculating means over areas.

Number marking in nouns, verbs, adjectives and pronouns was analysed. In the great majority of cases the lengths of morphemes marking a less marked category value were less than or equal to the one of morphemes marking a more marked category member. The results were especially clear for nouns and pronouns. The average difference in length between two values of the category of number is greater in the cases that support the hypothesis than in the few cases that run counter to it. There are more differences in segments than in syllables. Due to greater differences in frequency between singular and dual than between dual and plural or singular and plural, the result is most obvious for the difference between singular and dual. Here only two cases could be found which disprove the hypothesis (i.e. where the dual marker was shorter than the plural marker).

The present analysis shows that support for typological markedness in the category of number cannot only be found in morphological length but also in phonological length. It therefore supports the hypothesis that

zero marking can be a result of truncation due to the high frequency of a marker. The present study concentrated on overt coding and therefore on frequency induced effects, for example shortening of an existing marker of a less or unmarked category value. Cases in which a morpheme marking a more marked category value came into existence for iconic reasons are not the subject of the present study.
In the present study number marking by inner modification and umlaut was excluded for all bound number markers because it would have been impossible to determine the boundary between stem and affix. It is possible that by doing so the effect frequency has on structural coding was underestimated. This is because coding via umlaut or inner modification only does not lengthen the word and is therefore probably used predominantly in very frequent forms.
Another factor which was not investigated in this study is articulatory complexity of single segments. It is possible that some of the long markers of the less marked values additionally consist of articulatorily complex segments.

5 Acknowledgments

I would like to thank Bill Croft for introducing me to the concept of typological markedness, for many fruitful discussions on the topic of this paper and for commenting on various earlier versions of the paper. I am grateful to my reviewers Thomas Stolz, Bernd Kortmann and Christian Langstrof for their insightful comments. This work was supported by a grant of the DAAD.

References

Andrews, J. (1975). *Introduction to Classical Nahuatl.* Austin/London: University of Texas Press.

Asher, R. and Kumari, T. (1997). *Malayalam.* Routledge, London/New York.

Bromley, H. (1981). *A Grammar of Lower Grand Valley Dani.* Dept. of Linguistics, Research School of Pacific Studies, Australian National University.

Carlson, R. (1994). *A Grammar of Supyire.* Mouton de Gruyter, Berlin/New York.

Chapman, S. and Derbyshire, D. (1991). Paumari. In Derbyshire, D. C. and Pullum, G. K., editors, *Handbook of Amazonian Languages*, volume 3, pages 161–352. Mouton de Gruyter, Berlin/New York.

Childs, G. T. (1995). *A Grammar of Kisi.* Mouton de Gruyter.

Cole, D. (1955). *An Introduction to Tswana Grammar.* London Longmans and Co., London/Cape Town/New York.

Croft, W. (1996). 'Markedness' and 'Universals': From Prague School to Typology. In Jankowsky., K., editor, *Multiple Perspectives on the Historical Dimensions of Language*, pages 15–21. Nodus Publikationen.

Croft, W. (2003). *Typology and Universals.* Cambridge: Cambridge University Press.

Dayley, J. P. (1985). *Tzutujil Grammar.* Linguistics 107. University of California Press.

Dimmendaal, G. J. (1983). *The Turkana Language.* Dordrecht/Cinnaminson: Foris Publications.

Donohue, M. (1999). *A Grammar of Tukang Besi.* Mouton de Gruyter, Berlin/New York.

Dryer, M. (1989). Large linguistic areas and language sampling. *Studies in Language*, 13(2):257–292.

Dryer, M. (1992). The Greenbergian word order correlations. *Language*, 68(1):81–138.

Ebert, K. (1997). *A Grammar of Athpare.* Lincom Europa, München/Newcastle.

Everett, D. and Kern, B. (1997). *Wari: The Pacaas Novos Language of Western Brazil.* Routledge, London/New York.

Foley, W. (1991). *The Yimas Language of New Guinea.* Standford University Press, Stanford, California.

Fortescue, M. (1984). *West Greenlandic.* Routledge Kegan & Paul.

Frajzyngier, Z. and Shay, E. (2002). *A Grammar of Hdi.* Mouton de Gruyter, Berlin/New York.

Frantz, D. G. (1991). *Blackfoot Grammar.* University of Toronto Press, Toronto/ Buffalo/ London.

Galloway, B. (1993). *A Grammar of Upriver Halkomelem.* Linguistics 96. University of California Press.

Greenberg, J. (1966). *Language Universals: With Special Reference to Feature Hierarchies.* The Hague/Parin: Mouton & Co.

Hagman, R. (1977). *Nama Hottentot Grammar.* Bloomington: Indiana University.

Haspelmath, M. (2006). Against markedness (and what to replace it with). *Journal of Linguistics*, 42(1):25–70.

Haspelmath, M. (2008a). Frequency vs. iconicity in explaining grammatical asymmetries. *Cognitive Linguistics*, 19(1):1–33.

Haspelmath, M. (2008b). Reply to Haiman and Croft. *Cognitive Linguistics*, 19(1):59–66.

Haviland, J. (1997). Guugu Yimidhirr. In Dixon, R. and Blake, B. J., editors, *Handbook of Australian Languages*, volume 1, pages 26–180. John Benjamins, Amsterdam.

Holes, C. (1995). *Modern Arabic.* Longman, London/New York.

Jakobson, R. (1932). Zur Struktur des russischen Verbums. In Mathesius, V., editor, *Charistera Guglielmo Mathesio quinquagenario a discipulis et Circuli Pragensis sodalibus oblata.*, pages 74–84. Cercle Linguistique de Prague, Prague.

Jakobson, R. (1939). Signe Zéro. In *Mélanges de linguistique offerts à Charles Bally.*, pages 143–152. Geneva.

Kenesei, I., Vago, R., and Fenyvesi, A. (1998). *Hungarian.* Routledge, London/New York.

Kimball, G. and Abbey, B. (1991). *Koasati Grammar.* University of Nebraska Press, Lincoln/London.

Klamer, M. (1998). *A Grammar of Kambera.* Mouton de Gruyter, Berlin/New York.

Manelis Klein, H. E. (2001). *Toba.* Lincom Europa, München.

McGregor, D. and McGregor, A. (1982). *Olo Language Materials.* Dept. of Linguistics, Research School of Pacific Studies, Australian National University.

Merlan, F. (1994). *A Grammar of Wardaman.* Mouton de Gruyter, Berlin/New York.

Morris, G. W., Vyatyutnev, M. N., and Vokhmina, L. (1996). *Russian Face to Face. A Communicative Program in Contemporary Russian.* National Textbook Company, Lincolnwood, Illinois.

Müller-Ott, D. (1982). *Russische Grammatik.* Ott-Verlag, Tulln.

Neukom, L. (2001). *Santali.* Lincom Europa.

Osumi, M. (1995). *Tinrin Grammar.* University of Hawaii Press, Honolulu.

Payne, D. and Payne, T. (1990). Yagua. In Derbyshire, C. and K., G., editors, *Handbook of Amazonian Languages*, volume 2, pages 249–474. Mouton de Gruyter, Berlin/New York.

Press, I. (1986). *A Grammar of Modern Breton.* Mouton de Gruyter, Berlin/ New York/ Amsterdam.

Rau, D.-H. V. (1992). *A Grammar of Atayal.* Cornell University.

Roberts, J. (1987). *Amele.* Croom Helm, London/New York/Sydney.

Ruhlen, M. (1991). *A Guide to the World's Languages: Classification.* Stanford University Press.

Saltarelli, M. (1988). *Basque.* Croom Helm, London/New York/Sydney.

Sandalo, F. (1997). A grammar of Kadiwéu: with special reference to the Polysynthesis Parameter. *MIT Occasional Papers in Linguistics, Cambridge, Massachusetts*, 11.

Seegmiller, S. (1996). *Karachay.* LINCOM Europa, Munich/Newcastle.

Shixuan, X. (2001). *The Bisu Language.* Lincom Europa, München.

Stolz, T., Khizanishvili, T., and Levkovych, N. (2007). Lexikalische Duale. Typologische Gedanken zu den Übersetzungsäquivalenten von Deutsch *beide* in crosslinguistischer Sicht. *Lingua Posnaniensis*, 44:167–196.

Stolz, T., Stroh, C., and Urdze, A. (2006). *On Comitatives and Related Categories: A Typological Study with Special Focus on the Languages of Europe.* Mouton de Gruyter, Berlin, New York.

Stolz, T., Stroh, C., and Urdze, A. (2010). With(out). On the markedness relation between comitatives/instrumentals and abessives. *Word*, 58(2).

Terrill, A. (1999). *A grammar of Lavukaleve: A Papuan language of the Solomon Islands.* PhD thesis, Australian National University.

Trubetzkoy, N. (1931). Die phonologischen Systeme. *Travaux du Cercle Linguistique de Prague*, 4:96–116.

Trubetzkoy, N. (1939 [1969]). *Principles of Phonology.* (Translation of Grundzüge der Phonologie, Prague, 1939). Berkeley and Los Angeles: University of California Press.

Veselinova, L. (2005a). Suppletion in Tense and Aspect Categores. In Haspelmath, M., Dryer, M., Gil, D., and Comrie, B., editors, *World Atlas of Language Structures*, pages 322–325. Oxford University Press, Oxford Univ Press.

Veselinova, L. (2005b). Verbal Number and Suppletion. In Haspelmath, M., Dryer, M., Gil, D., and Comrie, B., editors, *World Atlas of Language Structures*, pages 326–329. Oxford University Press, Oxford.

Zúñiga, F. (2000). *Mapudungun.* Lincom Europa, München.

On the Status of [h]~[x] Alternations in German Dialects: The Case for Buccalization*

T. A. HALL

Abstract: The present article investigates German dialects with morphophonemic alternations between [h] and [x]. It will be shown that there are dialects with this regular alternation in which [x] in a coda must be derived from /h/ by a synchronic (non-assimilatory) process referred to below as 'Buccalization'. A cross-linguistic survey reveals that outside of Germanic non-assimilatory Buccalizations are clearly rare and possibly non-occurring. An analysis of Buccalization for German is proposed and the consequences of that analysis for rule-based and constraint-based theories are explored.

1 Introduction

A number of German dialects are attested in which morphemes exhibit regular alternations between the laryngeal [h] and the dorsal fricative [x]. A typical example (from the Southern Bavarian dialect described by Schatz, 1897, p.168) is presented in (1):

1. Alternation between [x] and [h]:

leih-en	[laihə]	'lend'
gelieh-en	[gli:hə]	'lent' (PAST PART)
lieh	[li:x]	'lent' (PRET)

Given the regularity of this type of alternation, the phonologists writing a synchronic grammar could presumably posit one of the two processes in (2):

* I would like to thank the two anonymous referees for their comments on an earlier version of the present paper and Bernd Pompino-Marschall for motivating me to undertake an investigation of Bavarian. An earlier version of sections 2.2 and 3 appeared in Hall (2009), which is being reproduced below with permission from the Franz Steiner Verlag.

2. Two possible synchronic rules:

(a) /x/ → [h]/ V __ V (Debuccalization)
(b) /h/ → [x]/ ___ # (Buccalization)

Rules which convert a sound like /x/ with an supraglottal articulation (like /x/) to a laryngeal like [h] are commonly referred to as Debuccalizations, while processes going in the opposite direction will henceforth be called Buccalizations.

In writing a synchronic analysis of dialects like the one in (1) one needs to decide whether or not one is dealing with a Debuccalization from /x/ or a Buccalization from /h/. It will be shown below that the German dialect in (1) does not give us the choice between (2a) and (2b) and that independent facts require one to posit Buccalization in (2b). This fact will be shown to be of significance because (non-assimilatory) synchronic Buccalizations like the one in (2b) appear to be otherwise unattested in the languages of the world.

The present article is organized as follows. In section 2 I present a brief survey of German dialects in which [h]~[x] alternations are completely regular and then present a more complete set of data from the dialect in (1). Section 3 discusses Debuccalizations and Buccalizations from the cross-linguistic point of view. There it will be shown that the former processes (i.e. 2a) are extremely common as synchronic processes, while the process in (2b) appears to be unattested (outside of Germanic). Section 4 discusses the consequences for phonological theory (both rule-based and constraint-based) of the process of Buccalization as a synchronic rule. It will be argued that [h] is phonologically a fricative (i.e. [-sonorant, +continuant]) and that Optimality Theory (OT) must allow for a constraint ranking which allows for Buccalizations as in (1b). That ranking will be shown to be problematic for the approach to OT proposed by De Lacy (2006), whose analysis predicts that there are no synchronic processes neutralizing place of articulation to dorsal (as in 2b). In section 5 I discuss the consequences of my analysis for the cross-linguistic facts. The conclusion is that, although Buccalizations are otherwise unattested cross-linguistically, the process does fulfill a phonological function in German dialects.

2 [h]~[x] alternations

This section consists of a brief survey of German dialects attested with morphophonemic alternations involving [h] and [x] (in section 2.1) followed by an in-depth discussion of these alternations in a single German dialect (i.e. the dialect in 1; see section 2.2). The material discussed below has been drawn from a number of the *Ortsgrammatiken* in the Neogrammarian tradition which have appeared as monographs in the past 120 years.

2.1 A brief survey of modern German dialects

It is now well established that the phoneme /h/ in Standard German has a highly limited distribution in the sense that it only surfaces (a) word-initially before a vowel (e.g. *Haus* [haʊs] 'house'), (b) intervocalically in a few non-native words (e.g. *Uhu* [uːhu] 'eagle owl', *Ahorn* [ahɔɐn] 'maple') and (c) between a consonant and a vowel in proper names (e.g. *Wilhelm* [vɪlhɛlm]). Note that the [h] in contexts (a)-(c) has in common that it is situated in syllable-initial position before a vowel. In other contexts (e.g. in coda position, as the final member of an onset cluster, syllable-initially before a consonant), [h] cannot occur (see Féry 2003 for discussion).

In contrast to Standard German, many regional varieties of German dialects contain *native* morphemes in which [h] surfaces intervocalically (i.e. context (b) referred to above). See, for example, the first two examples in (1) above. Since the [h] in these words is in stem-final position and since the following vowel is an inflectional suffix, it is possible to find alternants of the same stem with [x] in coda position; see the final example in (1).[1] In (3) I have provided an example of the verb conjugation for *fliehen* 'flee' in the Alemannic dialect of St. Gallen (Switzerland) described by Berger (1913, p.139-140). An examination of the stem-final consonant in each cell of this paradigm reveals that we are dealing once again with an alternation between [h] and [x].

1 Dialects with [h]~[x] alternations appear to be typical of Upper German (i.e. Bavarian or Alemannic). The first writer to my knowledge to observe that [h]~[x] alternations are a characteristic of the Bavarian dialect was Schmeller (1821, p.99). See also the discussion in Kranzmayer (1956, p.90-91) and Schirmunski (1962, p.365).

3. Verb conjugations in St. Gallen dialect:

INF.	flieh-en	[flyhə]
1 SG	flieh-e	[flyx]
2 SG	flieh-est	[flyxʃt]
3 SG	flieh-t	[flyxt]
1 PL	flieh-en	[flyhid]
2 PL	flieh-t	[flyhid]
3 PL	flieh-en	[flyhid]
PART PERF	ge-floh-en	[kflohə]

In (4) I have presented examples of an apparently regular [h]~[x] alternation in the Bavarian dialect of Zarz (from Lessiak, 1959, p.136-145).

4. Alternations between [x] and [h]:

Floh	[vloəx]	'flea'	p.139
Floehe	[vlehə]	'fleas'	p.138
hohe	[hoəhə]	'high ADJ ENDING'	p.138
hoch	[hoəx]	'high'	p.139

Lessiak (1959) notes at various points in his grammar (e.g. p.137, 197) that there are also suffixes which alternate between [x] and [h], although he does not always provide transcriptions.

The grammars from which the data in (3) and (4) have been taken do not present examples with [h]~[x] alternations in a systematic way; hence, it is difficult to tell whether or not we are dealing with a Debuccalization from /x/ or a Buccalization from /h/. This is not the case with the dialect presented earlier in (1). As I demonstrate in the following section the original source for that dialect (Schatz, 1897) provides a wealth of data which enables one to deduce the correct synchronic rule.

2.2 Imst German

In this section I present a larger set of examples illustrating [h]~[x] alternations from the dialect presented earlier in (1). This dialect can be classified as a regional variety of Southern Bavarian German. It is spoken in Imst, Austria (65 km west of Innsbruck) and was described in detail by

Schatz (1897). I refer henceforth to this variety as Imst German (IG).[2] IG [h] and [x] are both phonemic because they contrast in pre-vocalic position. Two representative examples are provided in (5a-b). In the former examples we see a minimal pair in which [h] and [x] surface between the diphthong [ɑi] and schwa. In the latter data set I have presented a near minimal pair in which the same segments surface between [ʀ] and schwa. In (5) and below I provide in the final column the page numbers from Schatz (1897) for all examples cited.

5. Contrast between [h] and [x]:

(a)	weihen	[wɑihə]	'consecrate'	p.176
	weichen	[wɑixə]	'soften'	p.99
(b)	Föhre	[foʀhə]	'pine'	p.106
	Birke	[piʀxə]	'birch tree'	p.99

The sound transcribed in (5) and below as [x] is described by Schatz (1897, p.9) as a voiceless fricative ('stimmloser Reibelaut'). In terms of place of articulation, IG [x] (as well as [k g]) are described as 'Gaumenlaute' (literally 'palatal sounds'), which in the case of [x], involves a constriction on the back part of the soft palate ('am hinteren weichen Gaumen'; p. 9). This description suggests that the sound in question is velar (i.e. IPA [x]) as opposed to uvular (IPA [χ]), but the exact place of articulation cannot be deduced from Schatz's description because he does not specify what he means by the 'back' of the soft palate. The present treatment does not crucially depend on whether or not [x] is phonetically velar or uvular because IG does not contrast velar and uvular sounds. Schatz (1897, p.9) describes [h] as an aspirate ('Hauchlaut'), which he distinguishes from true fricatives (i.e. 'Reibelaute') like [x].
Word-internal contrasts like the one in (5) are common in IG. By contrast, the data in (6) illustrate that in other environments, the contrast between [h] and [x] is suspended. In (6a) we can observe that [h] (and never [x]) occurs word-initially and in (6b) that [x] (and not [h]) surfaces

2 A larger corpus can be found in Schatz (1955), which includes material drawn from a number of regional Southern Bavarian dialects spoken in the Tyrolian area (including Imst). A description of IG eighty years after Joseph Schatz wrote his original grammar is Hathaway (1979).

word-finally. The final word in (6b) shows that IG has no process of Dorsal Fricative Assimilation converting [x] into a palatal allophone [ç] after front vowels, as in Standard German. The example in (6c) illustrates that only [x] (and never [h]) surfaces in coda position before an obstruent.

6. Contrast between [h] and [x] suspended:

(a)	Haus	[haus]	'house'	p.106
	Hanf	[hompf]	'hemp'	p.16
	hundert	[hundəʀt]	'hundred'	p.164
(b)	Buch	[puəx]	'book'	p.140
	reich	[ʀɑix]	'rich'	p.145
(c)	Docht	[dɔxt]	'wick'	p.39

In the following remainder of this section I consider the way in which [h] and [x] alternate in stem-final position when suffixes follow.
In (7a-h) I provide the three principal parts of several strong verbs whose infinitive stem ends in *h*. An inspection of the phonetic forms illustrates that these verb stems display alternations between [h] and [x]. The regularity of these alternations will be reinforced the additional examples provided below.[3]

7. Alternations between [x] and [h] in verbs:

(a)	leihen	[lɑihə]	'lend'	p.168
	geliehen	[gli:hə]	'lent (PAST PART)'	p.168
	lieh	[li:x]	'lent (PRET)'	p.168
(b)	seihen	[sɑihə]	'strain'	p.168
	gesiehen	[gsi:hə]	'strained (PAST PART)'	p.168
	sieh	[si:x]	'strained (PRET)'	p.168
(c)	zeihen	[tsɑihə]	'indict'	p.168
	geziehen	[tsi:hə]	'indicted (PAST PART)'	p.168
	zieh	[tsi:x]	'indicted (PRET)'	p.168

3 In contrast to other varieties of Bavarian German (see Merkle, 1986, p.53), *Präteritumschwund* had not affected IG at the time of the appearance of Schatz (1897); hence, we can observe in (7) and below the existence of overt preterit forms. Several examples in (7) exhibit alternations between [g]~[k]~ Ø in the past participle prefix (e.g. *geliehen* in 7a with [g] vs. *geflohen* in 7d with [k] vs. *gezogen* in 7e with Ø). These alternations will not be discussed below.

(d)	fliehen	[fliəhə]	'flee'	p.169
	geflohen	[kflouhə]	'flown (PAST PART)'	p.169
	floh	[flu:x]	'fled (PRET)'	p.169
(e)	ziehen	[tsiəhe]	'move'	p.169
	gezogen	[tsouhə]	'moved (PAST PART)'	p.169
	zog	[tsu:x]	'moved (PRET)'	p.169
(f)	sehen	[søihə]	'see'	p.172
	gesehen	[ksøihə]	'seen (PAST PART)'	p.172
	sah	[sɑ:x]	'saw (PRET)'	p.172
(g)	geschehen	[kʃøihə]	'happen'	p.172
	geschehen	[kʃøihə]	'happened (PAST PART)'	p.172
	geschah	[kʃa:x]	'happened (PRET)'	p.172
(h)	weihen	[wɑihə]	'consecrate'	p.76
	geweiht	[gwɑixt]/ [gwi:hə]	'consecrated (PAST PART)'	p.176
	weihte	[wi:x]/ [wɑihət]	'consecrated (PRET)'	p.176

On the basis of the examples like the ones in (7), I conclude that [x] surfaces in the coda and [h] in intervocalic position. This generalization is confirmed in the optional pronunciations for the final two examples under (7h): In these examples the dorsal fricative [x] surfaces in the first variant because it is in the coda and the laryngeal [h] in the second variant because it is between vowels.

Consider now the vowels adjacent to the [h] in the examples in (7). That the vowel following [h] in these words is always [ə] is simply a consequence of the fact that the inflectional suffixes of IG as in (7) are all schwa-initial. Some additional examples will be presented below in which a derivational suffix follows a stem-final [h] which contains a vowel other than schwa. The vowel which can occur to the left of [h]/[x] in the alternations in (7) and below is always long (or a diphthong). The non-occurrence of short vowels preceding [h]/[x] does not play a role in the analysis presented in section 4.

The same [h]~[x] alternation can be observed in inflected nouns and adjectives, as in the examples in (8a-l). In several of the examples presented below stem-final [h] can occur before a derivational suffix (e.g. the second item in 8k-l), which contains a vowel other than schwa.[4]

8. Alternations between [x] and [h] in nouns and adjectives:

(a)	Vieh	[fiːx]	'creature'	p.140
	Vieher	[fiːhəʀ]	'creatures'	p.140
	viehisch	[fiːhiʃ]	'brutish'	p.106
(b)	rauh	[ʀaux]	'rough'	p.152
	rauher	[ʀaihəʀ]	'rougher'	p.152
	rauhst	[ʀaixʃt]	'roughest'	p.152
(c)	hoch	[hoax]	'high'	p.152
	höchst	[heaxʃt]	'highest'	p.152
	höher	[heahəʀ]	'higher'	p.152
(d)	roh	[ʀoax]	'coarse'	p.152
	rohst	[ʀeaxʃt]	'coarsest'	p.152
	roher	[ʀeahəʀ]	'coarser'	p.152
(e)	schlau	[ʃlaux]	'sly'	p.152
	schlaust	[ʃlaixʃt]	'sliest'	p.152
	schlauer	[ʃlaihəʀ]	'slier'	p.152
(f)	scheuen	[ʃuihə]	'shrink from'	p.106
	scheu	[ʃuix]	'timid'	p.106
(g)	stolz	[waːx]	'proud'	p.106
	ein stolzer	[əwaːhəʀ]	'a proud (ADJ. ENDING)'	p.106
(h)	Bauch	[paux]	'abdomen'	p.106
	bauchig	[pauhig]	'bellied'	p.106
(i)	Pech	[pøix]	'pitch'	p.106
	verpechen	[fəʀpøihə]	'plaster up with pitch'	p.106
(j)	Blech	[pløix]	'metal sheet'	p.106
	blechener	[pløihəʀnəʀ]	'made of a metal sheet'	p.106
(k)	Milch	[milx]	'milk'	p.106
	milchig	[milhig]	'milky'	p.106
(l)	Kalk	[kxolx]	'lime'	p.106
	kalkig	[kxolhig]	'limy'	p.106

It can be observed that the fricative [x] in (8) surfaces consistently in the coda. The examples in (8a-j) illustrate that [h] occurs in intervocalic

4 Examples (8e-f) show that – in contrast to Standard German – the two stems *schlau* and *scheu* have a final consonant in IG (i.e. [h] or [x])

position after a (long) vowel. By contrast, the [h] in (8k-l) surfaces post-consonantally (i.e. after [l]; I have found no examples with [h] after [ʀ]). On the basis of the data in (7-8) I posit the following generalization concerning the distribution of [h] and [x] in alternating morphemes: The former sound occurs in pre-vocalic position and the latter sound in the coda.

It appears up to this point that the [h]~[x] alternations in (7-8) require either rule (9a) or (9b). The former is a Debuccalization and the latter a Buccalization.

9. Two possible synchronic rules:

(a)	IG-Debuccalization:	/x/→ [h]	/ __V
(b)	IG-Buccalization:	/h/→ [x]	/ in the coda

If IG-Debuccalization were correct, then alternating morphemes would have /x/, which then shifts to [h] before a vowel. By contrast, if one were to accept IG-Buccalization, the alternating morphemes would have /h/, which surfaces as [x] in the coda. The examples [waixə] and [piʀxə] from (5a-b) are important because they show IG-Debuccalization cannot be correct. Additional examples of stems ending in a non-alternating [x] have been given in (10a-e). In the pairs of words in this data set the stem ends in [x] regardless of whether or not a vowel-initial suffix follows. Note that the second word in each pair below contains [x] in prevocalic context, which is precisely the environment for [h] in (7-8).[5]

10. Non-alternating [x]:

(a)	Buch	[puəx]	'book'	p.140
	Bücher	[piəxəʀ]	'books'	p.140
(b)	Tuch	[tuəx]	'cloth'	p.140
	Tücher	[tiəxəʀ]	'cloths'	p.140
(c)	Mark	[moʀx]	'marrow'	p.141

5 Schatz (1897) makes it clear that there is no phonetic difference in IG between the non-alternating [x] as in (10) and the alternating [x] in (7-8). It would not be possible to analyze the dorsal fricative in (10) as a geminate and the same sound in (7-8) as a singleton because Schatz (1897, p.99) makes it clear that the geminate dorsal fricative [xx] only occurs intervocalically after short vowels.

	Marke	[mɑʀxəʀ]	'marrows'	p.141
(d)	reich	[ʀɑix]	'rich'	p.145
	reiche	[ʀɑixə]	'rich (ACC. MASC)'	p.145
(e)	weich	[woɑx]	'soft'	p.152
	weicher	[wɑixəʀ]	'softer'	p.152

The data in (10) tell us that IG-Buccalization in (9b) is the correct rule. This means that alternating [x] in in (7-8) requires an underlying /h/, while non-alternating [x] necessitates /x/. Representative examples of alternating and non-alternating morphemes can be seen in (11a-b) and (11c-d) respectively:

11. Underlying representations:

(a)	leihen	[lɑih-ə]	/lɑih-ə/	from 7a
	lieh	[liːx]	/liːh/	
(b)	fliehen	[fliəhə]	/fliəh-ə/	from 7d
	floh	[fluːx]	/fluːh/	
(c)	Tuch	[tuəx]	/tuəx/	from 10b
	Tücher	[tiəx̌əʀ]	/tiəx-əʀ/	
(d)	reich	[ʀɑix]	/ʀɑix/	from 10d
	reiche	[ʀɑixə]	/ʀɑix-ə/	

Morphemes with non-alternating [h] restrict the occurrence of that sound to word-initial position (see 6a) or word-internally before a vowel (see the first example in 5a and 5b). IG-Buccalization cannot affect the [h] in either context because it only affects an [h] in the coda.[6] On the basis of the data in Schatz (1897), it is clear that IG-Buccalization is a very regular process which affects every /h/ in the coda.[7] Since /h/ and /x/ are phonemic, IG-Buccalization is a neutralization because it suspends the

6 IG also displays very regular alternations between [w] and [b], which appear to have the same distribution as [h] and [x]: *freuen* [fʀœiwə] 'be pleased' p. 81, *ich freue* [ifʀœib] 'I am pleased' p. 81. Schatz (1897, p.81-82) is clear that the alternant with [b] occurs in final position and the one with [w] before a vowel. This type of alternation therefore requires either a rule converting /b/ into [w] before a vowel or one converting /w/ to [b] in the coda. See Hall (2009) for some discussion.

7 Two apparently idiosyncratic exceptions are *Truhen* [tʀuːh.nə] 'footlockers' (cf. *Truhe* [tʀuːhə] 'footlocker') and *Blahen* [ploːh.nə] 'linen (pl.)' (cf. *Blahe* [ploːhə] 'linen (sg.); p. 135).

lexical contrast between /h/ and /x/ to the latter sound in coda position. Note too that IG-Buccalization is non-assimilatory. The reason is that /h/ shifts to [x] in coda position regardless of whether or not the preceding sound is a front vowel, a back vowel, or a consonant.[8] [9]
The change from underlying /h/ to [x] in the coda cannot be analyzed as the part of a more general process of neutralization. This point can be illustrated with the examples in (12a-e), which consist of noun and verb stems ending in a consonant other than [h] or [x]. All of these examples have been presented in pairs to show that the stem-final consonants do not alternate. In the first word in each pair the stem-final consonant is situated in the coda and in the second word it is in the onset. The examples show that stops (12a), affricates (12b), fricatives (12c), nasals (12d) and liquids (12e) undergo no changes in syllable-final and syllable-initial position.[10]

12. Nouns and verbs with non-alternating stem-final consonants:

(a)	Lamm	[lomp]	'lamb'	p.141
	Lämmer	[lempəʀ]	'lambs'	p.141
	Zeit	[tsɑit]	'time'	p.139
	Zeiten	[tsɑitə]	'times'	p.139
	Rad	[ʀoːd]	'wheel'	p.141
	Räder	[ʀøidəʀ]	'wheels'	p.141

8 IG also has a synchronic process converting /h/ to [x] after [x] or [kx] in connected speech, e.g. *ich leihe her* [i laix xea] 'I lend' (cf. *her*) [hea] in isolation; see Schatz (1897, p.19). In contrast to IG-Buccalization in (9b), this cross-word process is obviously assimilatory.

9 In Hall (2009) I show that rule inversion (Vennemann, 1972b) transpired in IG. Put simply, this means that at an earlier stage in Germanic, there was a synchronic process of Debuccalization (as in 9a), which later on became inverted to IG-Buccalization in (9b). The reader is referred to Hall (2009) for details.

10 Word pairs like [ʀoːd]~[ʀøidəʀ] (among others) illustrate that IG has no rule of Final Devoicing as in Standard German. Schatz (1897, p.9) describes sounds like [p] and [b] as 'voiceless' ('stimmlos'), the difference being that [p] is fortis and [b] lenis. To my knowledge the only gaps involve [b] and [n]. There do not appear to be any examples with a surface [b] in the coda because this sound is in complementary distribution with [w] (recall note 6). Stems with [n] in coda position are difficult to find because [n] typically causes the preceding vowel to nasalize and then deletes if it is word-final, e.g. *Bahn* [poũ] 'train' (cf. *Bahnen* [poũnə] 'trains'; p.132). For discussion see Schatz (1897, p.94-97).

	Türke	[tiʀk]	'Turk'	p.127
	Türken	[tiʀkə]	'Turks'	p.127
	Auge	[oug]	'eye'	p.142
	Augen	[ougə]	'eyes'	p.142
(b)	Dampf	[tompf]	'steam'	p.74
	dämpfen	[tempfə]	'deaden'	p.74
	Schütze	[ʃits]	'marksman'	p.127
	Schützen	[ʃitsə]	'marksmen'	p.127
	falsch	[foltʃ]	'wrong'	p.152
	falscher	[føltʃəʀ]	'more wrong'	p.152
	Bäcker	[pøkx]	'baker'	p.127
	Bäcker	[pøkxə]	'bakers'	p.127
(c)	Hilfe	[hilf]	'help (SG.)'	p.132
	Hilfen	[hilfə]	'help (PL.)'	p.132
	Riese	[ʀiːs]	'giant'	p.127
	Riesen	[ʀiːsə]	'giants'	p.127
	Hirsch	[hiəʀʃ]	'stag'	p.128
	Hirsche	[hiəʀʃə]	'stags'	p.128
	arm	[oʀm]	'poor'	p.152
	ärmer	[øʀməʀ]	'poorer'	p.152
	Zeitung	[tsɑituŋ]	'newspaper'	p.133
	Zeitungen	[tsɑituŋə]	'newspapers'	p.133
(e)	Zahl	[tsoːl]	'number'	p.132
	Zahlen	[tsoːlə]	'numbers'	p.132
	Herr	[heɑʀ]	'gentleman'	p.127
	Herren	[heɑʀə]	'gentlemen'	p.127

The words in (12) with a dorsal, labial or coronal in the coda are important because they imply that IG-Buccalization cannot be reduced to a general neutralization of all fricatives (or all obstruents) to a dorsal sound. It can also be deduced that there is no general tendency in IG to convert stops and affricates into fricatives.

3 Buccalization and typology

The correct synchronic process of IG-Buccalization and the incorrect process IG-Debuccalization have been reproduced in (13):

13. (a) IG-Debuccalization: /x/→ [h]/ __V
    (b) IG-Buccalization: /h/→ [x]/ in the coda

The cross-linguistic literature reveals near unanimity that Debuccalizations like the one in (13a) are more 'natural' than Buccalizations, as in (13b). In the present section I discuss the typological evidence which has led phonologists to this conclusion.[11]
There is no doubt that Debuccalizations are common synchronic processes in the languages of the world. This impressionistic view is confirmed when one examines cross-linguistic surveys, e.g. Trigo Ferre (1988); Lavoie (1996, p.291); Lavoie (2001, p.39); Kirchner (2001, p.95); Fallon (2002, pp.123-202); Cser (2003), which include together a significant number of examples of Debuccalizations in which the output segment is [h].
Eleven synchronic Debuccalizations have been presented in (14). In the final column I have listed the respective languages, the country in which the language is spoken and the original sources. The list in (14) has been restricted to synchronic Debuccalizations in which the laryngeal [h] is the output. Thus, I have not included Debuccalizations in which the output is a glottal stop, e.g. /t/ surfacing as [ʔ]. Examples like the ones in (14) are easy to find and hence it would not be difficult to compile a much longer list.

14. Synchronic Debuccalizations creating [h]:

(a)	/p t k s/→ [h]/ __]$_\sigma$	(Tiriyó; Suriname; Parker (2001, p.110))
(b)	/p t k s/→ [h]/ __]$_\sigma$	(Macushi; Brazil, Guyana; Parker (2001, p.114))

11 It is not my goal in the present study to offer a formal definition of phonological 'naturalness'. Instead, I focus below on the rarity (and possible non-existence) of Buccalizations outside of Germanic. I provide some speculative remarks concerning the (un)naturalness of IG-Buccalization in section 5.

(c)	/s/→ [h]/__]$_\sigma$	(Malay; Malaysia; Durand (1987, p.87))
(d)	/s/→ [h]/__{C, #}	(Spanish dialects; Latin America; Lipski (1964, p.34))
(e)	/s/→ [h]/__#	(Lenakel; Vanuatu; Lynch (1978, p.9))
(f)	/k/→ [h]/__ (#) V	(Sye; Vanuatu; Crowley (1998, p.28))
(g)	/k/→ [h]/__ (#) V	(Toba Batak; Indonesia; Hayes (1986, p.478))
(h)	/t/→ [h]/__ #	(Liverpool English; England; Harris (1990, p.266))
(i)	/x/→ [h]/in the onset	(Hungarian; Hungary; Siptar and Törkenczy (2000, p.276))
(j)	/x/→ [h]/context unclear	(Paez; Columbia; Gerdel (1973, p.38))
(k)	/x/→ [h]/__ #	(Carrier; Canada; Story (1984, p.47))

The rules in (14) have in common that the input sound is a consonant with a supraglottal articulation (typically a voiceless fricative like /s/ or /x/) and that the output is [h]. The typical context is syllable- or word-final position, although other contexts are also attested.
The frequency of Debuccalizations can be contrasted with the complete lack of examples illustrating the mirror-image process of Buccalization. This point is confirmed by the cross-linguistic studies referred to above, i.e., Lavoie (1996, p.291); Lavoie (2001, p.39); Kirchner (2001, p.95); Fallon (2002, p.123-202); Cser (2003), which have no examples. Significantly, it is clear from these studies that the respective authors actually looked for Bucccalizations. To the point Lavoie (1996, p.304) writes: "There are...no examples of a glottal gaining an oral place in the data base." De Lacy (2006, p.355) makes an equally strong claim concerning non-assimilatory place neutralizations in synchronic rules: "[n]o language ever …neutralizes PoA [Place of Articulation] to dorsal…". It will be seen below that Lavoie's and De Lacy's observation that Buccalizations are not attested cross-linguistically has been taken as a given by a number of other linguists. Perhaps Larry Trask put it best of all

when he wrote in an email message of 11 July 1995 to the Linguist List http://www.linguistlist.org/issues/6/6-960.html in response to his own query concerning the possible existence of Buccalizations: "It really does look as if the glottal region is a vast sink from which no segment ever returns."

To summarize: Synchronic Debuccalizations are extremely common, while synchronic Buccalizations are unknown (outside of the Imst example). The paucity of Buccalizations requires some modification: It is not difficult to find languages in which [h] surfaces as a sound with a supraglottal articulation (like /x/) if that change is conditioned by an adjacent vowel. For example, according to Vago (1980, p.129) there is an allophonic process in Hungarian in which /h/ assimilates to [x] after a back vowel and to [ç] after a front vowel in final position or before a consonant. According to Hoijer's (1945), Navaho /h/ surfaces as [x] before [a], as [x^w] before [o], and as a 'frontal palatal' before [i e] (pp. 16-17). In Japanese (Ito and Mester, 2004, p.556), /h/ surfaces allophonically as the bilabial fricative [ɸ] before high back vowels and as [ç] before high front vowels. Similar processes affecting /h/ are attested in the Melanesian language Tinrin (New Caledonia; Osumi (1995, p.19-20)) and Carribean Spanish (Trigo Ferre, 1988, p.49).[12]

There are also languages on record in which /h/ assimilates to an adjacent consonant, e.g. in Toba Batak (Hayes, 1986, p.481) /h/ undergoes a total assimilation to a preceding obstruent (e.g. /marsap hita/ → [marsappita] 'let us smoke'). A similar type of assimilatory change is also attested in IG in connected speech, as pointed out in note 8.

By contrast, I claim that Buccalizations NOT triggered by an adjacent segment are not attested. Examples of these hypothetical changes are presented in (15).[13]

12 In Ifugao (Philippines; Newell (1956, p.529)) there is a synchronic process which converts /h/ to [s] after /i e/. This process is assimilatory if front vowels like /i e/ are coronal (Clements and Hume, 1995).

13 It is often assumed or argued that Buccalizations are unattested diachronic changes, e.g. Sturtevant (1945, p.2) states that "the...development of breathing to spirant is impossible." Campbell (1998, p.135) similarly writes that "... the change *k*>*h* is very common and not unexpected, whereas the change *h*- > *k*- is all but unknown." Vennemann (1972a, p.875) posits the hierarchy [x] >[χ]>[h]>Ø as "a universal of change", implying that languages can debuccalize (e.g. [χ]>[h]) but not buccalize. Howell (1991) is the only linguist to my knowledge who claims that "phonetic [h] can indeed develop

15. Regular synchronic processes which are unattested:

(a) /h/→ [x]/ __]$_\sigma$
(b) /h/→ [x]/ $_\sigma$[__
(c) /h/→ [s]/ __]$_\sigma$
(d) /h/→ [s]/ $_\sigma$[__

One could expand the list in (15) with Buccalizations in which the output is some segment other than [x] or [s], e.g.[t], [p].
Another apparent counterexample to the claim made in (15) can be seen in the Korean data in (16) from Iverson (1989, p.287-288). In (16a) it can be observed that /h/ surfaces in coda position as an unreleased coronal, i.e. [t˺]. The reason the change from /h/ to [t˺] is not a true Buccalization like the ones in (15) is that the process in (16a) is a very general one (referred to in the literature as Obstruent Neutralization). Obstruent Neutralization neutralizes ALL obstruents to either [p˺], [t˺] or [k˺] in the coda. For example, the same rule converts the two fricatives (/s, s'/), the three affricates (/č č^h č/) and the three stops (/t t^h t'/) to [t˺], the three labial stops (/p, p^h, p'/) to [p˺] and the three dorsal stops (/k, k^h, k'/) to [k˺]. An example illustrating the neutralization of /s/ to [t˺] can be seen in (16b).

16. Korean obstruent neutralization:

(a)	/čoh-ko/	[čot˺.k^{h}o]	'good and'
	/čoh-ɨni/	[čo.hɨ.ni]	'as (it is) good'
(b)	/os/	[ot˺]	'clothes'
	/os-ɨn	[o.sɨn]	'as for the clothes'

The Korean data are important because they show that /h/ cannot surface in the coda for one of two reasons: (i) [h] is a fricative and fricatives are not allowed in the coda, or (ii) [h] is aspirated ([+spread glottis]) and Korean does not allow this feature to surface in the coda. By contrast, the hypothetical processes in (15) refer to /h/ only.[14]

into a spirant [x] or [ç]" (pp. 92-93). The reader is referred to Hall (2010) for a critical analysis of Howell (1991).

14 Blevins (2004, p.160) discusses a synchronic process of Misantla Totonac, according to which ([+sonorant]) /h/ surfaces as the obstruent [ɬ] in the coda. As in Korean, this example does not involve a true Buccalization: /h/ cannot surface in the coda because Misantla Totonac imposes a strict ban on ALL sonorants in that context.

4 A phonological analysis of Buccalization

In the present section I discuss the features for [h] (in section 4.1) and then posit an OT analysis of IG-Buccalization (in section 4.2). In section 4.3 I consider the significance of my OT analysis for the current debate in the literature concerning place neutralizations.

4.1 Features for [h]

Given the regularity of the [h]~[x] alternations discussed above, I postulate that IG /h/ and /x/ are both voiceless fricatives which only differ in terms of place features. See Bessell (1992), who defends a similar position on the basis of the phonological behavior of /h/ in other languages. The features presupposed in my analysis are presented in the following matrices; '√' indicates the presence of a node in feature geometry[15]:

17. Distinctive features for /x/ and /h/ in IG:

	x	h
[sonorant]	—	—
[continuant]	+	+
[PLACE]	√	
[DORSAL]	√	

/h/ is analyzed here as a placeless segment in line with a number of studies on the phonology of laryngeals (e.g. Bessell, 1992; Rose, 1996). Given this treatment, the alternation in IG between [h] and [x] (see below) can be shown to involve the addition of place features only, while major class features ([sonorant]) and manner features ([continuant]) remain constant.[16]

15 My analysis makes no reference to the feature [consonantal] and hence I refrain from presenting that feature in (17) and below. In IG /h/ is the only laryngeal phoneme. Schatz (1897) does not discuss whether or not the dialect has [ʔ], as in Standard German. In any case the glottal stop is epenthetic and not underlying in the latter dialect, if not in all German dialects.

16 There are two conceivable approaches to laryngeal features. According to the first view, the distinctive laryngeal feature for IG is [voice]; hence, sounds like /b d g/ will be specified for the [LARYNGEAL] node and [+voice], while sounds like /p t k/, /x/ and /h/ are [LARYNGEAL] and [-voice]. According to the second view, the (privative)

A number of studies have discussed the analysis of laryngeals like /h/ in terms of major class and manner features (e.g. Chomsky and Halle, 1968; McCarthy, 1988; Bessell, 1992; Rose, 1996; Fallon, 2002). The analysis of /h/ as [–sonorant, +continuant] in (17) contrasts with the claim made in the literature for other languages that /h/ is phonologically a glide, i.e. [+sonorant] (in addition to [–consonantal]); see Chomsky and Halle (1968) and many subsequent writers. One of the arguments in favor of the latter featural analysis of laryngeals comes from the behavior of those sounds with respect to nasal harmony in languages like Malay. The analysis of /h/ as [+continuant] is also controversial; see, for example, McCarthy (1988, p.7-8) who writes "[f] or purely articulatory (or definitional) reasons, [h] and [θ] cannot carry distinctions for the feature [continuant] (or any other manner feature)."

In my view the correct analysis of laryngeals like /h/ is a language-specific fact. In languages like Malay it might very well be the case that /h/ is [+sonorant] if it behaves like a sonorant in the phonology. The same point holds for the non-specification of /h/ for [continuant] and other manner features in the languages McCarthy (1988) investigates. But in IG we have /h/ clearly patterning phonologically with the fricative /x/ and this fact justifies the features in (16). To the best of my knowledge no contradictory evidence from IG exists.

Given the features in (17), a hypothetical Debuccalization of /x/ to [h] (for the languages 14i-k) can be expressed in a rule-based framework as the deletion of the [PLACE] node (and its dependent [DORSAL]), as in (18a).[17] Given the approach in (18a), the mirror-image process of Buccalization is analyzed as the addition of [DORSAL] to a [–voice, –sonorant, +continuant] segment which lacks place features, as in (18b). I assume that node generation (Archangeli and Pulleyblank, 1994) guarantees that the addition of [DORSAL] will automatically trigger the addition of the place node.

---

feature [spread glottis] is the distinctive laryngeal feature; hence, sounds like /p t k/ (and /x h/) are [LARYNGEAL] and [spread glottis], while /b d g/ are unmarked for either feature. I adopt the first position below, even though it is not crucial to my analysis.

17 Formal analyses of Debuccalizations have been proposed in a number of theoretical frameworks, e.g. Dependency Phonology (Durand (1987) based on earlier work by Lass (1976)), Charm and Government Phonology (Harris, 1990, 1997), Feature Geometry (McCarthy, 1988; Fallon, 2002), and Optimality Theory (De Lacy, 2006).

18. A featural analysis of Debuccalization in (a) and Buccalization in (b):

a. [−voice, −sonorant, +continuant]]$_\sigma$

ǂ

[PLACE]

|

[DORSAL]

b. [−voice, −sonorant, +continuant]]$_\sigma$

¦

[DORSAL]

4.2 An OT analysis of IG-Buccalization

The OT analysis presented below is intended to account for the data from IG presented in section 2.2. In particular, the following three regularities will be captured: (i) IG-Buccalization occurs in coda position only, (ii) the output of IG-Buccalization is dorsal and not coronal or labial, (iii) the contrast between /x/ and /h/ is preserved word-internally. The analysis requires reference to the following constraints:

19.

(a) NO-CODA-h:	[h] is prohibited from surfacing in the coda
(b) MAX-PLACE:	No deletion of place features
(c) *LAB:	A labial is marked as ungrammatical
(d) *COR:	A coronal is marked as ungrammatical
(e) *DORS:	A dorsal is marked as ungrammatical
(f) *h:	[h] is marked as ungrammatical

The constraint in (19a) is a context-sensitive markedness constraint penalizing surface forms with [h] in the coda. The constraint is independently necessary in languages like IG (and other dialects of German), in which [h] only surfaces in the onset but not in the coda. See Féry (2003, p.231), who posits a very similar constraint in order to account for the distribution of Standard German [h]. The constraint in (19b) is a standard faithfulness constraint penalizing the deletion of place features. Given my treatment of /h/ as placeless, this constraint therefore penalizes output forms with [h] from /x/ as the input. In (19c-e) I have listed markedness constraints penalizing the three major places of articulation (see Lombardi 2002 and a number of other linguists). The constraint in (19f) (from Féry, 2003; Davis and Cho, 2003) penalizes words with a surface [h].

In tableau (20) I have presented a representative example of an IG word (from 8a) in which coda /h/ buccalizes to [x]. The high ranking constraint NO-CODA-h is necessary to eliminate the faithful candidate in (20a). The reason the output of Buccalization is the dorsal [x] and not the coronal [s] or the labial [f] can be achieved if *LAB and *COR outrank *DORS, as indicated below. I comment on the theoretical significance ranking of this constraint ranking in section 4.3 below.

(20) Input: /liːh/	NO-CODA-h	MAX-PLACE	*LAB	*COR	*DORS	*[h]
a. [liːh]	*!			*		*
b. → [liːx]				*	*	
c. [liːs]				**!		
d. [liːf]			*!	*		

(21) Input: /waix-ə/	NO-CODA-h	MAX-PLACE	*DORS	*[h]
a. [waihə]		*!		*
b. → [waixə]			*	

(22) Input: /laih-ə/	NO-CODA-h	MAX-PLACE	*DORS	*[h]
a. → [laihə]				*
b. [laixə]			*!	

Tableaux in (21) and (22) illustrate how the present analysis can account for the contrast between surface [x] and [h] in examples like the ones presented in (7h) vs. (11a). In the remaining tableaux I omit the two constraints *LAB and *COR because they are not relevant for the analysis. In the first tableau we see that MAX-PLACE must outrank *DORS so that the candidate with [x] can be selected. In the latter tableau the candidate with [h] wins because of the ranking *DORS» *[h]. In (23) and (24) we have contexts in which there is no contrast between [x] and [h], i.e. onset and coda respectively (recall the data in 6). The markedness constraint NO-CODA-h is playing a crucial role in the second tableau because it eliminates candidate (24b). Note too that if /h/ were interpreted as the input in (24) in conformance with Richness of the Base, then the correct winner in (24a) would also be selected.[18]

(23) Input: /haus/	NO-CODA-h	*DORS	*[h]
a. → [haus]			*
b. [xaus]		*!	

(24) Input: /puəx/	NO-CODA-h	*DORS	*[h]
a. → [puəx]		*	
b. [puəh]	*!		*

18 Tableau (23) presents an apparent problem given the Richness of the Base hypothesis. Since there is no contrast between [h] and [x] in word-initial position, one would expect my analysis to produce the correct output even if the input were /x/, i.e. /xaus/ for (23). The problem is that the intended winner [haus] incurs a fatal violation of MAX-PLACE, so that [xaus] is incorrectly selected. I do not see Richness of the Base forcing one to posit an input /x/ for word-initial position. In Standard German (in which the generalizations in 7 are the same as in IG), there are many loanwords beginning with [x] (or [ç]), which contrast with [h] (see Robinson, 2001, for discussion). Significantly, there is no evidence at all that any of the loanwords with [x] or [ç] reduce that fricative to [h]. The data from IG in section 2.2 have been obtained from Schatz (1897), but Schatz was not concerned with describing loanwords in IG. I hypothesize that there were IG loanwords with initial [x] (as in other varieties of German) which never reduced to [h]

4.3 Discussion

In the OT literature (see Hall 2010 in press, for a recent survey) there is a longstanding debate concerning place of articulation markedness. Simply put, there are two relevant questions: (a) Is it possible to identify one of the three major places of articulation (i.e. labial, coronal, dorsal) as least marked? And (b) Is place of articulation markedness universal or language-specific? The type of evidence discussed in the literature with respect to questions (a) and (b) has been drawn from a wide variety of properties, e.g. consonant epenthesis, inputs to place assimilations, frequency, acquisition and saliency.

The argument for place of articulation markedness relevant for the present paper is place neutralization. The literature cited below is in agreement that the output of place neutralization is an unmarked sound. Given this view, the process of place neutralization discussed above (i.e. IG-Buccalization) provides evidence that dorsal is less marked than labial or coronal because dorsal ([x]) is the output.[19] I contend that the unmarkedness of the dorsal place of articulation is a language-specific fact of IG and not universal; see Hume and Tserdanelis (2002), who espouse a similar view. We will see below that both of my claims conflict with some of the proposals made in the recent literature.

Languages which neutralize place of articulation to dorsal (as in IG) can be captured in an OT approach with a markedness hierarchy in which the constraint militating against dorsal is lower ranked than the ones militating against labial or coronal. This ranking (see 25a) is precisely the one proposed for IG in the preceding section. As shown earlier, the hierarchy in (25a) correctly selects a dorsal sound (i.e. [x] as the output of a place neutralization (in this case from /h/).

Two place hierarchies:

(a) *LABIAL, *CORONAL » *DORSAL » *[h]

(b) *DORSAL, *LABIAL » *CORONAL » *PHARYNGEAL

The hierarchy in (25a) for IG conflicts with approaches to OT which see coronal as the (universal) unmarked major place. According to that ap-

19 There is no independent evidence from IG to my knowledge (e.g. epenthesis, assimilation) that dorsal is the unmarked place.

proach, the unmarkedness of coronal with respect to labial and dorsal is captured with the universally fixed hierarchy in (25b); see Lombardi (2002) as well as Prince and Smolensky (2004, p.215).[20] I see the constraints in the hierarchy in (25a) as being freely rankable (depending on the language) and not universally fixed.

De Lacy (2006) proposes a universal markedness hierarchy which is similar to the one in (25b) in the sense that it sees coronal as being less marked than labial or dorsal. Place neutralizations are argued to have only two possible outputs, namely coronal and glottal. As pointed out in section 2, De Lacy (2006, p.355) makes a very clear prediction concerning the type of place neutralizations that are claimed to be NOT possible as synchronic rules: "[n]o language ever ... neutralizes PoA [Place of Articulation] to dorsal ..." De Lacy (2006) argues that the apparent cases of neutralization to dorsal that have been discussed in the literature (see Rice, 1996) can be explained in other ways; for example, in languages like Selayarese in which a multiple place contrast neutralizes in final position to the velar nasal [ŋ], De Lacy (2006) argues that the sound transcribed as '[ŋ]' is really glottal. In other cases (e.g. in Oceanic), there is a neutralization of /t/ to [k], but De Lacy (2006) claims that this change is always historical and never synchronic.

The data presented in section 2.3 from IG pose a clear counterexample to De Lacy's claim concerning impossible place neutralizations. The neutralization from /h/ to [x] is synchronic (as opposed to the Oceanic example mentioned above). What is more, the output cannot be interpreted as 'glottal', because it is clearly dorsal.[21]

My analysis of IG is supported by the treatment of place assimilation in Sri Lankan Portuguese Creole proposed by Hume and Tserdanelis (2002). Those authors show that various criteria for markedness (e.g. place assimilation) point to the unmarkedness of labials in that language. They argue that there is a hierarchy of place of articulation constraints which is similar to the one proposed above in (25a) in the sense that the

20 Lombardi (2002) posited her hierarchy in (25b) primarily on the basis of epenthesis, although it is clear that she intends for the markedness relations in her hierarchy to capture other phenomena as well, e.g. place neutralization. The constraint *PHARYNGEAL in (25b) refers to laryngeal sounds like [h]. That constraint serves a similar function to the constraint *[h] in my hierarchy in (25a).

21 See also Rice (2008) for criticisms of De Lacy (2006). The former author points to Manam as a language which neutralizes a multiple place contrast to labial.

constraints are argued to be freely rankable depending on the language and not universally fixed, as in (25b). One of the predictions made in this approach is that there should be languages in which dorsal is the unmarked place. The one example Hume and Tserdanelis (2002, p.454) cite illustrating the unmarkedness of dorsal as the trigger of place assimilation if Chukchi. The analysis of IG above provides support in the form of place neutralization for dorsal unmarkedness.

It has been observed that place neutralizations to dorsal only involve nasals (Selayarese) or stops (Oceanic; Blevins (see 2004)). The materials presented from IG above are significant because they show that it is also possible to have a fricative undergoing place neutralization to dorsal.[22]

5 Conclusion

The present article has investigated a German dialect (Imst German, IG) with regular alternations between [h] and [x] which require that the latter sound be derived from the former one by a non-assimilatory neutralization (IG-Buccalization). It was argued that the data require /h/ to be analyzed as a fricative (i.e. [-sonorant, +continuant]) and that the major class and manner class features for /h/ can differ from language to language. In terms of OT, Buccalization was argued to require a ranking in which the markedness constraint militating against dorsal sounds (*DORS) is ranked lower than the constraints penalizing coronals (*COR) or labials (*LAB). This analysis was shown to be problematic for universally fixed hierarchies which situate the constraint *COR lower than *LAB and *DORS.

I conclude this article with a speculative note. It was shown above that IG-Buccalization appears to be unique in the languages of the world. If this is the case, why do we have it in German?

IG-Buccalization has a clear phonological motivation. As noted earlier,

22 According to an anonymous reviewer, the analysis for IG posited above is problematic because it goes contrary to the "generally accepted universal that coronal segments are universally less marked" than labials or dorsals. As pointed out by a number of researchers mentioned above (summarized in Hall 2010, in press), there are simply too many examples of rules which are problematic for the claim that coronal is the least marked place. In my view the burden of proof now lies on the shoulders of those linguists who believe that coronal is universally the unmarked place.

in both Standard German and IG, the sound [h] has a limited distribution in the sense that it only surfaces syllable-initially before a vowel. Any native speaker of German feels that words with a syllable-final surface [h] are simply foreign. For this reason, morphemes in IG which end in /h/ need to alter this sound on the surface if they are not followed by a vowel-initial suffix. One way of doing this would be to delete the /h/ in syllable-final position, but German (including IG) only allows for a limited number of segmental deletions. It is no doubt for this reason that IG chooses to retain the major class and manner features for /h/ in the output and to only alter the place features. Note that this functional explanation is accounted for in the formal OT analysis in tableau (20), but that the functional explanation does not tell us why IG wants the output to be [x] as opposed to [s] or [f]. One could speculate that [h] is acoustically closer to [x] than the other voiceless fricatives, but this is a question that needs to remain open for future research.

The analysis of IG makes an implicit prediction with respect to typology. If IG-Buccalization makes phonological (and perhaps phonetic) sense, then the absence of Buccalizations in other languages is probably accidental. There should be no principled reason why there could not be languages with similar Buccalizations, provided that they are phonologically motivated. I therefore leave open for further research a thorough, typological study of alternations between [h] and other sounds (e.g. [x], [s], [f]). This type of investigation is important because it would tell us whether or not these alternations require Buccalizations and if so, what the output is.

References

Archangeli, D. and Pulleyblank, D. (1994). *Grounded Phonology.* MIT Press, Cambridge.

Berger, J. (1913). Die Laute der Mundarten des St. Galler Rheintals und der angrenzenden vorarlbergischen Gebiete. In *Beiträge zur Schweizerdeutschen Grammatik 3*, pages 1–231.

Bessell, N. (1992). The typological status of /ʔ, h/. *CLS*, 28:56–71.

Blevins, J. (2004). *Evolutionary Phonology: The Emergence of Sound Patterns.* Cambridge University Press, Cambridge.

Campbell, L. (1998). *Historical Linguistics. An Introduction.* Edinburgh University Press., Edinburgh.

Chomsky, N. and Halle, M. (1968). *The Sound Pattern of English.* Harper and Row, New York.

Clements, G. and Hume, E. (1995). The Internal Organization of Speech Sounds. In Goldsmith, J., editor, *The Handbook of Phonological Theory*, pages 245–306. Blackwell, Oxford.

Crowley, T. (1998). *An Erromangan (Sye) Grammar.* University of Hawaii Press, Honolulu.

Cser, A. (2003). *The Typology and Modelling of Obstruent Lenition and Fortition Processes.* Akadémiai Kiadó, Budapest.

Davis, S. and Cho, M. (2003). The distribution of aspirated stops and /h/ in American English and Korean: an alignment approach with typological implications. *Linguistics*, 41(4):607–652.

De Lacy, P. (2006). *Markedness: Reduction and Preservation in Phonology.* Cambridge University Press, Cambridge.

Durand, J. (1987). On the Phonological Status of Glides: The Evidence from Malay. In Anderson, J. and Durand, J., editors, *Explorations in Dependency Phonology*, pages 79–107. Foris Publications, Dordrecht.

Fallon, P. (2002). *The Synchronic and Diachronic Phonology of Ejectives.* Routledge, New York.

Féry, C. (2003). Onsets and Nonmoraic Syllables in German. In Féry, C. and van de Vijver, R., editors, *The Syllable in Optimality Theory*, pages 213–237. Cambridge University Press, Cambridge.

Gerdel, F. (1973). Paez phonemes. *Linguistics*, 104:28–48.

Hall, T. A. (2009). Rule inversion in a regional variety of Bavarian German. *Zeitschrift für Dialektologie und Linguistik*, 76:137–164.

Hall, T. A. (2010). *Directionality in Historical Linguistics: Are Diachronic Buccalizations Attested?* Ms. Indiana University.

Hall, T. A. (2010 in press). Coronals. In van Oostendorp, M., Ewen, C., Hume, E., and Rice, K., editors, *Companion to Phonology*. Blackwell, Oxford.

Harris, J. (1990). Segmental complexity and phonological government. *Phonology*, 7(2):255–300.

Harris, J. (1997). Licensing inheritance: An integrated theory of neutralisation. *Phonology*, 14.3(3):315–370.

Hathaway, L. (1979). *Der Mundartwandel in Imst in Tirol zwischen 1897 und 1973*. W. Braumüller, Wien.

Hayes, B. (1986). Assimilation as spreading in Toba Batak. *Linguistic Inquiry*, 17(3):467–499.

Howell, R. (1991). *Old English Breaking and its Germanic Analogues*. Niemeyer, Tübingen.

Hume, E. and Tserdanelis, G. (2002). Labial unmarkedness in Sri Lankan Portuguese Creole. *Phonology*, 19(3):441–458.

Ito, J. and Mester, A. (2004). The Phonological Lexicon. In McCarthy, J., editor, *Optimality Theory. A Reader.*, pages 552–568 [Excerpt from Ito, J. & Mester, A. (1999) The Phonological Lexicon. In: N. Tsujimura (ed.) The Handbook of Japanese Linguistics. Oxford, Blackwell, 62–100]. Blackwell, Oxford.

Iverson, G. (1989). On the category supralaryngeal. *Phonology*, 6(2):285–303.

Kirchner, R. (2001). *An Effort Based Approach to Consonant Lenition*. Garland, New York.

Kranzmayer, E. (1956). *Historische Lautgeographie des Gesamtbairischen Dialektraumes*. H. Böhlau, Wien.

Lass, R. (1976). *English Phonology and Phonological Theory: Synchronic and Diachronic Studies*. Cambridge University Press, Cambridge.

Lavoie, L. (1996). Consonantal strength: results of a data base development project. *Working Papers of the Cornell Phonetics Laboratory*, 12:207–232.

Lavoie, L. (2001). *Consonantal Strength. Phonological Patterns and Phonetic Manifestations*. Garland, New York.

Lessiak, P. (1959). *Die deutsche Mundart von Zarz in Oberkrain*. Elwert Verlag, Marburg N.G.

Lipski, J. M. (1964). On the weakening of /s/ in Latin American Spanish. *Zeitschrift für Dialektologie und Linguistik*, 51.1:31–43.

Lombardi, L. (2002). Coronal epenthesis and markedness. *Phonology*, 19(2):219–251.

Lynch, J. (1978). *A Grammar of Lenakel*. The Australian National University, Canberra.

McCarthy, J. (1988). Feature geometry and dependency: A review. *Phonetica*, 43:84–108.

Merkle, L. (1986). *Bairische Grammatik*. Hugendubel, München.

Newell, L. (1956). Phonology of the Guhang Ifugao dialect. *Philippine Journal of Science*, 85(4):523–539.

Osumi, M. (1995). *Tinrin Grammar.* University of Hawaii Press, Honolulu.

Parker, S. (2001). On the phonemic status of [h] in Tiriyó. *International Journal of American Linguistics*, 67(2):105–118.

Prince, A. and Smolensky, P. (2004). *Optimality Theory. Constraint Interaction in Generative Grammar.* Blackwell, Malden.

Rice, K. (1996). Default variability: The coronal-velar relationship. *Natural Language and Linguistic Theory*, 14(3):493–543.

Rice, K. (2008). Markedness in Phonology. In de Lacy, P., editor, *The Cambridge Handbook of Phonology*, pages 79–97. Cambridge University Press, Cambridge.

Robinson, O. (2001). *Whose German? The ach/ich Alternation and Related Phenomena in Standard and Colloquial.* John Benjamins Publishing Company, Amsterdam.

Rose, S. (1996). Variable laryngeals and vowel lowering. *Phonology*, 13(1):73–117.

Schatz, J. (1897). *Die Mundart von Imst. Laut-und Flexionslehre.* KJ Trübner, Strassburg.

Schatz, J. (1955). *Wörterbuch der Tiroler Mundarten.* Wagner, Innsbruck.

Schirmunski, V. M. (1962). *Deutsche Mundartforschung: Vergleichende Laut- und Formenlehre der deutschen Mundarten.* Akademie Verlag, Berlin.

Schmeller, J. (1821). *Die Mundarten Bayerns: Grammatisch dargestellt.* K. Thienemann, München.

Siptar, P. and Törkenczy, M. (2000). *The Phonology of Hungarian.* Oxford University Press, Oxford.

Story, G. (1984). *Babine and Carrier Phonology: A Historically Oriented Study.* Summer Institute of Linguistics, Arlington, Texas.

Sturtevant, A. (1945). Notes on Gothic morphology. *Publications of the Modern Language Association of America*, 60:1–2.

Trigo Ferre, L. R. (1988). *The Phonological Derivation and Behavior of Nasal Glides.* PhD thesis, MIT.

Vago, R. (1980). *The Sound Pattern of Hungarian.* Georgetown University Press, Washington.

Vennemann, T. (1972a). Phonetic detail in assimilation: Problems in Germanic phonology. *Language*, 48:863–892.

Vennemann, T. (1972b). Rule inversion. *Lingua*, 29:209–242.

On the Gradual Understanding of Legal Texts in the Process of Reading - Resistance Strategies during Text Comprehension?

RAINER DIETRICH
JULIA HILLEBRAND
YVONNE STAKIC

Abstract: The following article investigates subjects' comprehension of technical texts. Our main question is whether inferences are automatically formed in the process of text comprehension. To answer this, we measure eye movements during reading. The results of our trials are not consistent with the so-called minimalist hypothesis of inference. Comparing processing times of simple everyday texts with those of legal texts yields significant evidence to support the conclusion that readers form deep inferences even while processing difficult material.

1 Background

Successfully reading and comprehending a text involves a series of cognitive steps. These steps form two distinct groups based on their content and type. Researchers have investigated many factors that influence the course and result of the process, in particular the properties of the text and (to a much lesser extent) the prerequisites of the reader; see, for instance, the comprehensive introduction by Ballstaedt et al. (1981). The first of these two groups of steps encompasses those that process the information contained *within the text*. The second group encompasses the steps that connect the text information with information *outside the text*. Together, this information constitutes the reading situation and the reader's general knowledge.

The situation model of Kintsch and Van Dijk (1978) for instance, describes the process of reading comprehension as an AI-system that combines levels of symbolic representations with higher perception based representations. It assumes that knowledge is not only symbolically represented in the form of variously complex information units, but that an internal model of the state of affairs described in the text is represented as well. The propositional representation serves as the basis for the construction of the mental model. The propositional representation also enriches, refines, and partly modifies the mental model through the processing of world knowledge.
Following the work of Kintsch (Kintsch, 1988, 1989), researchers refer to the results of the first group of steps as "the text basis" and to the results of the second group of steps as the "situation model". The goal of Kintsch's construction integration theory is to model conceptual inferences during text comprehension. In his model, world knowledge interacts explicitly and in detail with text information.
Reading comprehension is understood as a constructive and interpretive process, whereby the meaning of the text is built step by step integrating textual information, world knowledge, expectations, and convictions. Elaborating on the proposition units of the text, this model extends to so called situations containing text-related events, actions, persons, and episodes.[1]

2 Question

This paper investigates an observation concerning a special case of inferring from the second group of processing steps. Under what conditions

1 And God said, let there be light: and there was light. The universe's genesis was obviously brought about by oral communication and oral communication still prevailed in the Greek societies of the fifth and fourth centuries b.c. Extremely skillful texts like the Odyssey originate in oral communication - until they were written down. Today they are almost buried in oblivion. Our contribution to this Festschrift strives to lay the ground for a revival of oral communication of extended texts. Why should repeated listening to the oral version of, say, the wording of a law not guarantee a deeper understanding than reading its written version? We strongly believe that Bernd Pompino-Marschall is the personality to tackle the unorthodox project and design and run an empirical investigation testing for this intriguing hypothesis. Here we make a submission of the written part of such a comparative analysis.

are global inferences triggered during reading? An inference refers to the activation of information not explicitly expressed in the text. The task for researchers has been to determine the inferences that take place during reading (i.e., online) and the particular circumstances that accompany them.

For a while now, there have been two dominant inference models in discussion. The first dominant inference model is the minimalist approach. According to the minimalist hypothesis (McKoon and Ratcliff, 1988), only easily accessible inferences are formed automatically during reading. These include, for example, inferences that contribute to text coherence (i.e. that assist pronoun comprehension) or simple bridging inferences (i.e. causal relationships that can be quickly and easily retrieved from long-term memory). McKoon and Ratcliff call these kinds of inferences "local inferences". More complicated inferences are formed during normal reading situations (those without specific comprehension goals) only when:

1. There is a significant gap between consecutive semantic units; or

2. There is a contradiction between consecutive semantic units.

Automatic minimalist inferences help initiate so-called strategic processes, which form the basis for additional text comprehension. In particular, these strategic processes include inferences at the conceptual level, i.e., easily accessible inferences and concepts of action that play a role in local text coherence.

The second dominant inference model is the constructivist approach. According to this view (Kintsch, 1988), so-called global inferences in addition to local inferences are formed automatically and online during reading, even when no specific comprehension goals exist. Global inferences link disparate propositions and concepts by retrieving information from long-term memory. In particular, the constructivist model addresses the variety of processes involved in inference formation. In the construction phase, a semantic representation of new text information is produced and linked to thematically related concepts in the reader's general world knowledge, resulting in a semantic network between the two. However, this semantic network also contains information not required for text comprehension. A further step, the integration phase, is thus needed to convert the elaborated and incoherent information produced in the construction phase into a coherent network. This takes place through the repeated activation of specific concepts in the reader's general world knowledge. These concepts, reinforced through repeated activation, become a part of the final semantic network, at which point they can be regarded as inferences.

3 Forming inferences while processing difficult texts

3.1 The BBAW study

Our investigation was initiated based on the conclusions of a study by the interdisciplinary research group "Sprache des Rechts: Vermitteln, Verstehen, Verwechseln" of the Berlin-Brandenburg Academy of Sciences and Humanities (BBAW) (Becker and Klein, 2008). The group's over-arching task was to understand how prior knowledge affects the comprehension of complicated texts. The texts consisted of long and difficult legal texts. Due to the nature of the texts, this study can be considered on the whole ecologically more relevant than those with short texts, as has been the case in most previous studies. The subjects of the BBAW study participated in a role-playing game in which they had to solve a problem based on their comprehension of a text. The following sections of the General Terms and Conditions of Insurance (Allgemeine Versicherungsbedingungen, AVB) of the so-called Riester pension were crucial for solving this problem:
§6 Wann können Sie Ihre Versicherung ruhen lassen?

1. Sie können Ihre Versicherung vor dem vereinbarten Rentenbeginn jederzeit zum Schluss des laufenden Versicherungsjahres, bei Vereinbarung von Ratenzahlungen (vgl. §3 Ziffer 2) auch innerhalb des Versicherungsjahres zum Schluss eines jeden Ratenzahlungsabschnitts, ruhen lassen (Beitragsfreistellung). In diesem Fall setzen wir die versicherte Rente auf eine beitragsfreie Rente herab. Die beitragsfreie Rente wird nach den anerkannten Regeln der Versicherungsmathematik für den Zeitpunkt der Beitragsfreistellung

errechnet. Der aus Ihrer Versicherung für die Bildung der beitragsfreien Rente zur Verfügung stehende Betrag mindert sich um einen Abzug. Der Abzug beträgt 0,2 Prozent der Differenz zwischen dem zum vereinbarten Rentenbeginn vorhandenen Deckungskapital * 3) und dem zum Zeitpunkt der Beitragsfreistellung vorhandenen Deckungskapital * 3). Sofern gebildetes Kapital *1) gemäss §9 für eine Verwendung als Altersvorsorge-Eigenheimbetrag ausgezahlt wurde, wird dies bei der Berechnung der beitragsfreien Rente berücksichtigt. Eine Übersicht der garantierten beitragsfreien Renten ist im Versicherungsschein enthalten.

2. Ihre Versicherung können Sie nach einer Beitragsfreistellung jederzeit durch Fortsetzung der Beitragszahlung wieder in Kraft setzen. Hierfür findet der bei Abschluss des Vertrages gültige Tarif Anwendung.

§6 Can I suspend my insurance?

1. *You can suspend your insurance (i.e., suspend payments) before the agreed starting date of your retirement at any time after the termination of an insurance year. When paying by instalments (see sec. 3 para. 2), you can suspend your insurance during the insurance year at any time after the end of an instalment payment period. If you do suspend your insurance, we will lower the insured pension to a non-contributory pension. The non-contributory pension is calculated for the period of payment according to the normal rules of insurance mathematics. The amount from your insurance available for a non-contributory pension decreases by one deduction equal to 0.2 % of the difference between coverage capital available at the agreed starting date of your retirement *3) and the coverage capital available at the beginning of payment suspension *3). Capital *1) according to sec. 9 cashed for old-age/retirement home provisions payment will be factored in to the calculation of the non-contributory pension. The insurance policy contains an overview of the guaranteed non-contributory pensions.*

2. *After suspending payment, you may put into effect your insurance at any time by resuming payments. The tariff valid stipulated in your contract will apply.*

§7 Wann können Sie Ihre Versicherung zur Auszahlung des Rückkaufswertes kündigen?

1. Sie können Ihre Versicherung vor dem vereinbarten Rentenbeginn jederzeit zum Schluss des laufenden Versicherungsjahres, bei Vereinbarung von Ratenzahlungen (vgl. §3 Ziffer 2) auch innerhalb des Versicherungsjahres zum Schluss eines jeden Ratenzahlungsabschnitts, schriftlich kündigen. Nach Kündigung erhalten Sie den Rückkaufswert.

2. Kündigen Sie Ihre Versicherung, so wird gemäss §176 Versicherungsvertragsgesetz der Rückkaufswert nach den anerkannten Regeln der Versicherungsmathematik für den Kündigungstermin als Zeitwert Ihrer Versicherung berechnet, wobei derselbe Abzug erfolgt, der bei einer Beitragsfreistellung nach §6 Ziffer 1 vorgenommen würde. Beitragsrückstände werden hierbei berücksichtigt. Bei beitragsfreien Versicherungen wird kein Abzug vorgenommen. Sofern gebildetes Kapital *1) gemäss §9 für eine Verwendung als Altersvorsorge-Eigenheimbetrag ausgezahlt wurde, wird dies bei der Berechnung des Rückkaufswertes berücksichtigt.

3. Der Rückkaufswert erreicht mindestens einen bei Vertragsabschluss vereinbarten Garantiebetrag, dessen Höhe sowohl vom Kündigungstermin als auch vom Zeitpunkt der Einstellung der Beitragszahlung abhängt. Eine Übersicht der garantierten Rückkaufswerte plus Überschussbeteiligung ist im Versicherungsschein enthalten.

4. Nach Beginn des Rentenbezugs ist eine Kündigung zur Auszahlung des Rückkaufswertes nicht mehr möglich.

5. Die Rückzahlung der Beiträge können Sie nicht verlangen.

§7 When can I cancel my insurance to cash the surrender value?

1. *You can cancel your insurance before the agreed starting date of your retirement at any time after the termination of an insurance year. When paying by instalments (see sec. 3 para. 2), you can cancel your insurance*

during the insurance year at any time after the end of an instalment payment period. After cancellation you will receive the appropriate surrender value.

2. *Should you cancel your insurance, the surrender value shall be calculated according to the normal rules of insurance mathematics for the cancellation date as the current value of your insurance (in accordance with sec. 176 of insurance policy code), minus the same deduction (sec. 6 para. 1) that applies for the suspension of insurance payment. Arrears in payment will be factored in as well. In the case of non-contributory insurance, no deduction shall occur. Capital *1) according to sec. 9 cashed for old-age/retirement home provisions payment will be factored in to the calculation of the surrender value.*

3. *The surrender value totals at least the agreed guarantee amount in the insurance contract. This amount depends on the cancellation date as well as on the date the payments are suspended. An overview of the guaranteed surrender values plus surplus contribution can be found in the insurance policy.*

4. *After you begin to draw the pension funds, you may no longer cancel the insurance to cash out the surrender value.*

5. *You may not demand the repayment of contributed sums.*

A particularly striking finding of this study was that subjects tended to arrive very early at an interpretation of concepts and propositions, which they maintained throughout the rest of their reading, even when the text explicitly called for a different interpretation. This suggests that the interpretation of new propositions and concepts is tied to ideas developed from previous ones. If a concept or proposition is understood incorrectly from the beginning, it will still be activated again later, but the already established understanding will not be questioned, even when the text clearly presents refuting evidence. The findings of the BBAW study do not square with either of the two inference models discussed above. For one, they directly contradict the constructivist assumption that global inferences are formed during normal reading (Kintsch, 1998, p.103). But they also challenge the minimalist view that additional inferences are formed when there is a contradiction between consecutive semantic units in the text (McKoon and Ratcliff, 1992, p.440). The findings of the BBAW suggest the presence of revision resistance, according to which previous interpretations are not revised even when strong evidence to the contrary shows them to be recognizably false. The objective of our study is to subject this explanation to a more exacting experiment.

3.2 Hypothesis

From the findings of the BBAW study, the following hypothesis can be derived:

In the case of difficult texts, non-automatic global inferences do not occur even when the text requires them.

This hypothesis is noteworthy insofar as it is compatible with neither of the two dominant inference models of text comprehension.

3.3 Operationalization

If this hypothesis is correct, then we can expect that the reader of a difficult technical text will not form global inferences, even if they are required by the specification of a comprehension task. One type of global inference occurs when the reader associates a word with a new concept after encountering textual information that is no longer consistent with the word's previous association (McKoon and Ratcliff, 1992, p.441). If the expected conceptual adaptation does not take place, then it can be assumed that the corresponding inferences do not take place either.

Research on eye movement during reading has shown that readers fixate longer on difficult passages than they do on easy ones, thus devoting greater amounts of visual attention to certain parts of the text. Since the reinterpretation of a lexical item requires additional cognitive effort, one can predict it to be accompanied by an increase in processing time. We should note, however, that processing time is also affected by other factors as well (Rayner, 1998; Rayner and Liversedge, 2004), such as word length, word frequency, ambiguity and others; their influence must, accordingly, be controlled experimentally.

3.4 Material

Our study consisted of six experimental texts (difficult) and six control texts (easy). For the experimental texts, we used passages from the AVB, as in the BBAW study described above. The control texts are from general-interest science texts used in the reading comprehension sections of the OECD Programme for International Student Assessment study (PISA; cf.Prenzel (2006) and in several school textbooks). The texts are between four and six sentences long and range from 58 to 78 words. The number of syllables per text ranges from 96 to 138. Below are samples of each text.

1. Experimental text:
Kündigen Sie Ihre Versicherung, so erfolgt ein Abzug. Gemäß Paragraph 176 Versicherungsvertragsgesetz wird der Wert Ihrer Versicherung, den Sie bei Kündigung ausbezahlt bekommen, nach den anerkannten Regeln der Versicherungsmathematik berechnet.
Der Abzug beträgt 0,2 Prozent der Differenz zwischen dem zum vereinbarten Rentenbeginn vorhandenen Deckungskapital und dem zum Zeitpunkt der Kündigung vorhandenen Deckungskapital. Lässt man die Versicherung vorher ruhen, erfolgt kein Abzug.

If you cancel your insurance a deduction shall occur. In accordance with sec. 176 of the insurance contract code, the value of your insurance cashed on cancellation is calculated according to the normal rules of insurance mathematics. The deduction is equal to 0.2 % of the difference between the coverage capital available at the agreed starting date of your retirement and the coverage capital available at the beginning of cancellation. If you have already suspended the insurance, no deduction shall occur.

2. Control text:
Ein Atom besteht aus einer Schale und einem Kern. Der Kern enthält unter anderem Protonen. Das sind kleine Teilchen mit einer positiven elektrischen Ladung. Die Protonen können wir mit kleinen Planeten vergleichen, die sich ständig um eine Achse drehen. Die sozusagen auf dem Proton befindliche positive Ladung rotiert dabei natürlich mit. Eine sich bewegende elektrische Ladung nennt man elektrischer Strom.
An atom is composed of an electron cloud and a nucleus. Protons make up one

part of the nucleus. Protons are small particles with a positive charge. A proton can be likened to a small planet perpetually revolving on its axis. The positive charge rotates along with the proton. A moving charge is called an electric current.

These texts were ordered into six pairs with each pair containing one experimental text and one control text. The two members of each pair were matched for length of utterances, word length, and word frequency. As discussed above, the processing of a text does not run uniformly for each section, sentence, and phrase. Phrases that contain already mentioned information are processed faster than those with new information. To keep with the hypothesis and to minimize variation, the observation was directed toward the focus phrase of the texts. Details are explained below. For this reason, each text was broken into proposition-length segments (clauses) with tagged topic and focus phrases.

3.5 Procedure

The six text pairs were randomly arranged into groups of three. One group was presented to each subject so that every subject received three experimental texts and three control texts. A group of 12 subjects made up of students and persons with non-academic backgrounds participated in the study, all of whom were paid for their participation. To exclude text-specific prior knowledge, subjects were selected with no background in law or insurance. In addition, none of the subjects wore glasses or contact lenses, so as to avoid sources of interference during eye position recording. Eye tracking was carried out with an SMI Eye Link 1. After the instructions were given and the eye-tracker was fitted and calibrated, the experiment began. Subjects were seated in front of a computer. When they pressed the space key, one of their assigned texts appeared on the screen in its entirety and the Eye Link began recording eye movements at a frequency of 50 Hz.
After completing a text, subjects had to answer multiple-choice questions about what they read. Subjects needed around 40 minutes to complete the three pairs of texts and questions. No specific problems with the texts nor the procedure were reported by the participants in the short closing interviews at the end of the sessions.

3.6 Data

3.6.1 Raw data

For the data to be admissible, reading times had to reflect a normal reading process, which was defined as a successive skipping of the eyes from left to right across the text, with the occasional regressive movement. Data from trials in which saccades occurred across the entire text or that contained longer gaps in recording were rejected. Data from 10 of the 12 subjects could be evaluated. In the case of one subject, there was an unexplained gap in the recording. Another subject was nervous, causing his eyes to skip irregularly across the screen.
In total, the reading times of the focus segments from 30 experimental texts and 30 control texts were analyzed. These 60 texts produced 254 data values for the experimental texts and 319 data values for the control texts. The discrepancy in data values between the experimental and control texts resulted from the varying number of focus segments in the text.

3.6.2 Standardization

There are reading time differences in the raw data that cannot be traced back to design factors alone. For one, not all the measured focus phrases were the same length. Some contained more words or phonologically more complex words, while others contained fewer or simpler words. To exclude this variance, the mean reading time was determined per syllable for each focus phrase. For another, it is well known that reading speed can vary from individual to individual. Since there were no reading speed screenings before the experiment, we determined the mean reading time per syllable for each subject and adjusted each trial according to a person-specific factor calculated from the quotient of the mean reading time per syllable and the mean reading time for the entire sample. All the data contained in the presentation and evaluation have been standardized in this way.

3.7 Results and evaluation

A set of 504 standardized reading times (= mean syllable reading times corrected per person) could be evaluated, 252 from experimental texts and 252 from control tests (see Table 1). Given the within-subjects design (ten subjects, three texts each) a paired t-test was administrated.

Table 1. Reading times, group means, and standard deviation of the experimental and the control data.

Groups	Nr. of stand. reading times	Total (ms)	Mean reading times total (ms)	SD
Experimental texts	252	42116	168	140.95
Control texts	252	33888	135	92.77
Paired, 2 sided t-test	p = 0.00221			

Reading times for the experimental condition, i.e. the more difficult text samples, are significantly longer than the control text reading times.

4 Discussion

According to the 'revision resistance' hypothesis, we predicted that readers of the experimental texts would fail to make global inferences triggered by conceptual reinterpretations. We expected, instead, to find similar reading times for both the experimental texts and the control texts. The analysis shows, however, that the reading times of the experimental texts and the control texts deviate significantly from one another ($p<0.01$, two-sided test). These results refute our hypothesis. Table 1 also shows that the unexpected difference results from a cause different from what we originally presumed. It is true that according to our hypothesis the reading times between control and experimental texts will vary. But the data shows that the relevant fixation times on focus phrases of the experimental texts are longer, not shorter, than the fixation times on the comparable parts for the control texts. This means that, contrary to our hypothesis, the subjects spent more time reading the experimental texts than they did reading the control texts.

Comparing the reading times for focus and topic segments of the experimental texts yields, however, a less convincing picture. It even seems to point into the opposite direction. Focus segments contain new information, while topic elements contain old or known information. Processing focus segments requires linking new concepts with old and/or known information. If this new information cannot be directly linked to the already known information, the reader must reactivate information already stored in the long-term memory or access information using world knowledge (i.e., through the formation of inferences). This cognitive processing takes time, which leads one to expect longer observation times for the focus segments (Starr et al., 2002, p.127). The comparison does, however, not yield significantly longer reading times for focus segments than for topic segments (Mann-Whitney U-test, two sided; normal distribution: $z = 1.057$; $p = 0.2904$). This result might, then, also be seen as indirect evidence in favour of the revision resistance hypothesis: Global inferences were not formed because subjects read over important and complex information without triggering global inferences. This argument is supported by the fact, that there is only one obvious evidence for an in depth inference. Among the experimental texts, text 1 stands out with the longest reading times. The reason for that is that the last focus segment seems to have occupied subjects particularly long; cf. table 2.

Table 2. Reading times experimental text no. 1.

Subject	Number of syllables	Total reading time (ms)	Mean reading time/syllable total (ms)	Mean reading time subject (ms)	Reading time last syllable (ms)
2	137	22098	161.30	149.63	391.60
3	137	23260	169.78	151.11	288.00
4	137	26344	192.29	162.18	628.56
5	137	29305	213.91	156.19	524.52
8	137	19262	140.60	147.69	461.12

The reason for this is probably the first mention of a new concept in the last section ('Abzug' engl.: *deduction*) which the readers then had to connect with the previous text, either by reactivating information already stored in their long-term memories or by connecting the new con-

cept with their world knowledge (inference formation). Being the only clear evidence in favour of the existence of global inferences, it might also be taken as evidence in favour of the revision resistance hypothesis. McKoon und Ratcliff exclude global inferences in developing their minimalist theory. They hold the view that inferences are formed automatically only when they are quick and easily accessible or important for local coherence. Global inferences, they argue, result from longer processes and from those formed by means of goal-oriented strategies (McKoon and Ratcliff, 1992, p.440). Kintsch, by contrast, admits automatic global inferences in his construction-integration model.
Review of the questionnaires, at last, reveals that, for all subjects, control text questions were easier to answer than experimental text questions. Interestingly, the slow readers made fewer mistakes, which suggests that their slow reading speed increased their reading retention. It must be noted, however, that the questionnaire results cannot be used to verify our hypothesis. Their sole purpose was to guarantee the difference between the control items and the experimental items.
Evaluation of all the data (reading times as well as questions about text comprehension) leads us to three important conclusions:

1. The revision resistance hypothesis cannot be maintained. The fixation times on the focus segments of the experimental texts are significantly longer than those of the control texts. This suggests that, contrary to our predictions, readers did not resist making revisions.

2. Readers did not take significantly less time to process the topic segments of the experimental texts than they did to process the focus segments of the experimental texts. This finding was unexpected.

3. The experimental texts were not comprehended as well as the control texts. Below we discuss possible causes for these results. First we consider the revision resistance hypothesis proposed by the BBAW study. Then we will consider possible sources of error in our own study.

4.1 Problems with the BBAW study

If the results of our experiment are regarded as correct, one might infer that the revision resistance hypothesis of the BBAW study is unfounded. The BBAW study, which examined the comprehension of legal texts, showed only a single case where the reader revised a false interpretation. In all other cases, subjects did not revise their false interpretations even when later passages explicitly gave them reason to do so. It was thus determined that in difficult technical texts non-automatic, global inferences are not formed even when they are motivated. The conclusions of the BBAW study are mostly based on data collected by means of the think-aloud method, whereby subjects speak their thoughts and feelings during the cognitive processing - simultaneously with the comprehension process, as it were. The purpose of the method is to investigate a subject's thought processes and to uncover problems in dealing with particular objects or texts (Kluwe, 1988, p.362). Ericsson and Simon (1993), following Kluwe (1988, p.326), discussed this method extensively in the 1980s, conceiving on its basis a general model for information processing. A central assumption of the think-aloud method is that subjects verbalize the contents of their short-term memory. According to Ericsson and Simon's general model, those short-term memory contents are composed of information immediately regarded and needed for further processing (Kluwe, 1988, p.362). In the BBAW study, subjects read a sentence and said what they understood by it. They were told not to simply repeat the sentence word for word - but just that what they comprehended.

It is possible that the think-aloud method does not make the actual inference processes sufficiently accessible. Other studies have criticized the validity of the verbalizations. Subjects do not express all the knowledge used with regard to a concept or proposition; in some cases, they state unnecessary knowledge as well. Kluwe questions whether think-aloud protocols are valid reports of cognitive events, and he raises the possibility of unconscious cognitive processes (Kluwe, 1988, p.369). If this criticism is legitimate, it may explain the inconsistency of our results with those of the BBAW study. Yet despite longer fixation durations, our readers did not comprehend the experimental texts as well as the control texts. This may be because they did indeed resist revising a previous interpretation, and thus failed to develop a deeper understanding of the text. Such an explanation is suggested by the reading observations in the BBAW study. The number of "reading repetitions" with lay subjects reported by Becker et al. (2004, p.49, fig. 9.1.6.) is significantly fewer than the number of reading repetitions with expert subjects (lawyers and insurance agents). That expert subjects read passages more than once and skipped backwards into the text more frequently than lay subjects did should not be taken to mean that lay subjects understood the text correctly the first time through; it only means that the lay subjects passed over conflicting information without trying to integrate it into their prior state of knowledge. But this interpretation is contested by the fact that lay subjects in general spent much more time reading than lawyers and insurance agents did (Becker et al., 2004, p.48-49, fig. 9.1.5.) which tells against the assumption that lay subject quickly passed over hard-to-integrate text segments. The questionnaire data of the BBAW study points in the same direction: in their answers to the difficult texts, lay subjects (comparable to those of our study) showed a better understanding than experts (Becker et al., 2004, p.238).

4.2 Methodological problems of our study

In the previous section, we discussed the possibility that the results of our study were unexpected because findings of the BBAW study were incorrect. An alternative explanation is that the findings of the BBAW study are correct but our results are not, possibly due to methodological problems.

4.2.1 Incorrect operationalization

Our assumption that the longer fixation times for readers of the experimental texts is not related to the formation of deep inferences might be wrong, as the longer fixation times may be caused by other cognitive processes during reading as well. Of course, constructivist theory claims that deep inferences can indeed be formed automatically (Rickheit and Strohner, 2003, p.567) and can hence influence fixation times at relevant text segments, creating a multi-phase process of inference formation. Yet it is precisely such a multi-phase process that might account for the longer fixation times. One can assume that the construction phase - in which a semantic representation of newly acquired text information is produced and linked to related concepts in the reader's world knowledge - runs for the most part automatically, and thus exerts little influence on the reader's cognitive ability. During the subsequent integration phase, however, various concepts in the semantic network must be converted from text segments and reader knowledge into a coherent network through cyclic merging of new input into active situation models. This processing phrase could bring about longer fixation times not due to inferences. This assumption is supported by questionnaire data showing that the experimental texts were not comprehended as well as the control texts. The lack of difference between the topic and the focus fixation times in the experimental texts might also support this explanation. However, the opposite explanation works for these results as well, namely, that they result from the automatic inference procedure rather than from the absence of inferences.

4.2.2 Problems with the texts

An introspective comparison of the difficulty of the test and control texts suggests that the control texts were too simple. This in turn might have shortened the reading times for the entire processing to the extent that the propositional comprehension of the experimental texts alone (without any deep inferences) lasted longer than the complete processing of the control texts. If, in keeping with the BBAW theory, no deep inferences were formed, then their absence would not have been noticed during the control texts, as their familiarity would allow for quick processing, even with inferences. The control texts - taken from the reading comprehension section of the PISA study and basic textbooks - were edited for a younger target group than the university students and educated adults in the study. The evaluation of the questionnaire also supports this conclusion. In the case of two control texts, 12 and 8, there were no wrong answers. In total, there were only 8 wrong answers to the control text questions, while there were 19 for the experimental texts. One reader answered 7 questions correctly, answering only one question of the experimental texts correctly but all six of the control texts. The questionnaire results can be explained in another way, however. It could be that, unlike the control texts, the subjects did not form global inferences when processing the experimental texts. And as the BBAW study already shows, the longer reading times can also be explained by the lack of familiarity with legal and insurance concepts.

5 Summary

After detailed review and discussion of the experiment results, we have found nothing to contest the experiment's conclusions. The fact that the results of our study are not consistent with those of the BBAW study can ultimately be explained by the difference in tasks. In the BBAW study, subjects took part in a role play in which they were asked to solve a problem by reading a text, namely, giving advice based on certain contractual provisions to a person who can no longer meet his or her regular insurance payments. In our experimental study, the task was different; our subjects were only asked to read texts in a concentrated fashion so that afterward they could answer questions about their contents. It is well known that the cognitive processing of the text during reading is linked to the given task and the comprehension goal. But this connection makes it hard to explain why readers who are given a problem to solve read the text more superficially, as it were, than when given the task to understand the text in its entirety. For the time being, we will thus maintain the view that the results of the BBAW study can either be attributed to the additional burden accompanying the think-aloud method (as a special case of double processing), or arose because the think-aloud method does not permit actual inferences manifest themselves.

References

Ballstaedt, S., Mandl, H., Schnotz, W., and Tergan, S. (1981). *Texte Verstehen, Texte Gestalten.* Urban & Schwarzenberg, Munich.

Becker, A. and Klein, W. (2008). *Recht verstehen: Wie Laien, Juristen und Versicherungsagenten die "Riester-Rente" interpretieren.* Akademie Verlag GmbH, Berlin.

Becker, A., Parádi, Z., and Witzmann, F. (2004). *Wie ist das nun wieder gemeint? Empirische Untersuchung zum Verstehen eines Verbraucherwerbtrages durch Laien und

Experten. Forschungsbereich der Interdisziplinären Arbeitsgruppe "Sprache des Rechts" der Berlin-Brandenburgischen Akademie der Wissenschaften, Berlin.

Ericsson, K. and Simon, H., editors (1993). *Protocol Analysis: Verbal Reports as Data (Rev. ed.)*. Cambridge: MIT Press.

Kintsch, W. (1988). The role of knowledge in discourse comprehension: A construction-integration model. *Psychological Review*, 95(2):163–182.

Kintsch, W. (1989). The Representation of Knowledge and the Use of Knowledge in Discourse Comprehension. In Dietrich, R. and Graumann, C. F., editors, *Language Processing in Social Context*, pages 185–209. Elsevier.

Kintsch, W. (1998). *Comprehension: A Paradigm for Cognition*. Cambridge University Press, Cambridge.

Kintsch, W. and Van Dijk, T. (1978). Toward a model of text comprehension and production. *Psychological Review*, 85(5):363–394.

Kluwe, R. (1988). Methoden der Psychologie zur Gewinnung von Daten über menschliches Wissen. In Mandl, H. and Spada, H., editors, *Wissenspsychologie*, pages 359–385. Psychologie-Verlag-Union, Munich.

McKoon, G. and Ratcliff, R. (1988). Contextually relevant aspects of meaning. *Journal of Experimental Psychology: Learning, Memory, and Cognition*, 14(2):331–343.

McKoon, G. and Ratcliff, R. (1992). Inference during reading. *Psychological Review*, 99(3):440–466.

Prenzel, M. (2006). *PISA 2006: Die Ergebnisse der dritten internationalen Vergleichsstudie*. Waxmann Verlag, Münster.

Rayner, K. (1998). Eye movements in reading and information processing: 20 years of research. *Psychological Bulletin*, 124:372–422.

Rayner, K. and Liversedge, S. (2004). Visual and Linguistic Processing during Eye Fixation in Reading. In Henderson, J. and Ferreira, F., editors, *The Interface of Language, Vision, and Action – Eye Movements and the Visual World*, pages 59–104. Psychology Press, New York.

Rickheit, G. and Strohner, H. (2003). Inferenzen. In Rickheit, G., Herrmann, T., and Deutsch, W., editors, *Psycholinguistics: An International Handbook*, pages 566–577. Mouton de Gruyter, Berlin.

Starr, M., Kambe, G., Miller, B., and Rayner, K. (2002). Cognitive Processes and Eye Movements during Reading. In Witruk, E., Friederici, A. D., and Lachmann, T., editors, *Basis Functions of Language, Reading, and Reading Disability*, pages 121–136. Kluwer Academic Publisher, Boston.

Influence of Smoking on Age Estimation from Voice

RALF WINKLER*

Abstract: Listeners are able to judge a speaker's age with reasonable accuracy based on listening to recorded speech samples. Different acoustic characteristics seem to be particularly affected by anatomical, physiological and psychological changes underlying the normal aging process. Age, however, is not the only factor affecting these parameters. Other speaker characteristics, for instance smoking, may have an influence on the same acoustic parameters. If the intersection of acoustic parameters coding age as well as smoking habit is large, the interrelation between these two perceptual qualities should be large too. To gain insight into the relation between these two perceptual qualities, speech samples of 24 young and elderly smoking and non-smoking adult women were recorded. Listeners were then asked to estimate the age and to judge the smoking habits of each speaker. In this study listeners performed very well in estimating age (i) and tobacco consumption (ii) independently of each other. Age estimations were not strongly influenced by speakers' smoking habits (iii), but the speakers' age influenced the perceived smoking habits significantly (iv). Since listeners were able to successfully interpret signs of age and signs of tobacco consumption (i and ii), the two perceptual qualities exist independently. Given (iv), there seems to exist a set of acoustic features indicating advanced age as well as increased smoking. There are probably additional acoustic cues guiding listeners in estimating age. Contrarily, lack of remaining features signalling smoking habits may force the listeners to use the subset features, resulting in judgments of smoking habits influenced by the speakers' age.

1 Introduction

Previous research has shown that listeners are able to estimate the age of a speaker quite accurately based on listening to recorded speech (Ptacek and Sander, 1966; Shipp and Hollien, 1969; Ryan and Burk, 1974). Hence a set of acoustic features exists that signal a speaker's age. Several voice

* When you changed from the ZAS to the Humboldt University formally, it was hard to get an appointment with you. Later on, after I left the ZAS, things became even harder. At that time, we arranged to meet ... as I remember, Thursday early in the morning to complete our work on the α-β model ... some colleagues were very jealous of our weekly appointment at that time!

quality features like fundamental frequency (F_0), jitter, shimmer and spectral tilt as well as temporal features like segment durations (hence tempo) and pauses have been identified as markers of chronological and perceived age (for details see Linville, 2001). These acoustic characteristics probably result from anatomical, physiological, and psychological changes in speech production and perception emerging during adulthood.

The accuracy of age estimation is usually defined as some relation (Shipp and Hollien, 1969; Ryan and Burk, 1974; Hartman, 1979; Neiman and Applegate, 1990) or difference between chronological and perceived age (Neiman and Applegate, 1990; Braun and Cerrato, 1999). This accuracy primarily depends on the characteristic acoustic and temporal features in the speech signal. It has been shown (Schötz, 2006; Winkler, 2009) that accuracy rates decline progressively when listeners judge age from spontaneous speech, reading samples, single words, phonated vowels and whispered vowels. As fewer acoustic cues are present in a stimulus, listeners' accuracy declines. However, previous work has shown that a number of other factors influence listeners' judgment of age as well. Some of these factors relate to specific listener and speaker characteristics. Another variation observed in listeners' judgment of age (i.e. centralisation) does not have a clear source.

A quite strong effect frequently described in the literature is the centralisation of age judgments. Listeners typically overestimate the age of younger and underestimate the age of elderly speakers (Shipp and Hollien, 1969; Hartman, 1979; Shipp et al., 1992; Schötz, 2005; Winkler, 2009). Differences in sex and age between listeners and speakers have been discussed as possible reasons for misestimation of age in Hollien and Tolhurst (1978). These factors, however, failed to explain the perceptual data observed in subsequent studies, where age and sex differences were made comparable. Despite the lack of a clear explanation this effect is consistently present in age estimations from recorded voice samples.

Relatively small influences on accuracy have been found for listener characteristics. Achieved accuracy (here in terms of percent correctly classified stimuli) was higher for the young compared to the elderly listeners (Linville and Korabic, 1986; Jacques and Rastatter, 1990). In Huntley et al. (1987), middle aged adults were superior to young and elderly listeners. Another interesting result regarding listener characteristics, namely no difference between listener groups, was described in Braun (1996), where experts with extensive experience in the forensic analysis of anonymous voices performed comparable to university students with no particular training in auditory phonetics.

Somewhat stronger influences on listener accuracy have been found for a number of speaker characteristics. Regarding a speaker's sex, in some studies accuracy was higher for female voices compared to male voices analyzed in the context of read speech (Neiman and Applegate, 1990) and single words (Schötz, 2006). In Schötz (2006), however, accuracy was comparable for female and male speakers when analyzing continuous speech samples. Up to now, results suggest that any effect of a speaker's sex on accuracy is moderate at best. Another speaker factor with almost no influence on accuracy is the speaker's first language. The achieved accuracies for American (Ptacek and Sander, 1966; Linville and Fisher, 1985; Linville and Korabic, 1986; Neiman and Applegate, 1990), German (Braun, 1996; Brückl and Sendlmeier, 2003; Winkler, 2009), Swedish (Schötz, 2006), Italian (Braun and Cerrato, 1999), and Japanese (Nagao, 2006) speakers are comparable as long as speakers and listeners share the first language. Conflicting results have been obtained when listeners do not know the language of the speaker: Nagao (2006) found lower accuracy for non-native listeners, but Braun and Cerrato (1999) did not. Scenarios like this need more studies to determine the influence on accuracy. A further impact on accuracy was suggested in Stölten and Engstrand (2002) for dialect colouring of speech, because they found a strong positive correlation between perceived age and perceived dialectal strength. A speaker's health was found to have a rather strong influence on accuracy. In Kreul and Hecker (1971), listeners were able to estimate the age quite accurately for healthy speakers, but this was not the case for subjects affected by laryngeal cancer. Similarly, heavy smokers obtained higher perceived age values compared to non-smokers of comparable chronological age based on read speech in Braun (1996).

Laryngeal cancer (Kreul and Hecker, 1971) and extensive tobacco consumption (Gilbert and Weismer, 1974) have a notable effect on laryngeal structure and function. Therefore, it is likely that laryngeal cancer (Hecker and Kreul, 1971) as well as heavy smoking (Gilbert and Weismer, 1974; Verdonck-de Leeuw and Mahieu, 2004) influence acoustic parameters, for instance mean fundamental frequency (F_0), maximum rate of change of F_0, and F_0 perturbations. If these parameters are part of the set of acoustic features signalling a speaker's age then accuracy of age estimations would be affected by these speaker characteristics.

In fact, parameters like fundamental frequency (Honjo and Isshiki, 1980; Stoicheff, 1981; de Pinto and Hollien, 1982; Mueller, 1997; Linville, 2001), as well as voice perturbation measures, namely jitter (Orlikoff and Baken, 1990; Xue and Deliyski, 2001) and shimmer (Orlikoff, 1990) show typical variations as a function of speaker age. Moreover, studies on the perceptual relevance of acoustic and temporal features in age estimation have found that listeners use voice quality parameters (Winkler and Sendlmeier, 2006; Winkler, 2007b), especially features of F_0 (Shrivastav et al., 2003; Harnsberger et al., 2006; Schötz, 2006; Winkler, 2007a). In women, fundamental frequency lowers with advanced age (Linville, 1996; Decoster and Debruyne, 2000; Baken, 2005; Harrington et al., 2007; Nishio and Niimi, 2008) and listeners seem to be sensitive to this acoustic characteristic (Linville and Fisher, 1985; Linville, 1987; Winkler, 2007b) by judging talkers to be older with decreasing pitch.

Fundamental frequency is probably only one of a whole set of acoustic parameters which might be used by listeners to judge smoking habits and age. Rather than evaluating the impact of acoustic features on listener judgments, the main objective of this study was to analyze the influence of speakers' smoking habits on the perceived age in healthy adult women. Braun (1996) observed a small increase of perceived age in heavy smokers around an age of 40 years as opposed to non-smokers comparable in age.

In the current study very young and rather elderly adults were used to find out, whether similar effects could be observed in age ranges where the perceptual centralisation effect acts strongest. In this study, perceived age and perceived smoking habits were determined. As both perceptive qualities were determined independently, it was possible to additionally relate these qualities to each other. Unlike Braun, who used read speech to determine perceived age, in this study single words were used. The reason for using rather short stimuli with simple linguistic structure was to facilitate the search of the acoustic features guiding listeners in estimating age and judging smoking habits in subsequent studies. In this study interactions between age estimation and judgment of smoking habits were interpreted and conclusions were drawn regarding the perceived age and perceived smoking habits of women in early and late adulthood.

2 Data and methods

2.1 Speakers

The speech corpus contained recordings of 24 female speakers. Fifteen recordings originate from a database previously collected by the author (Winkler, 2009) for the purpose of studying the acoustic and temporal characteristics of young and elderly voices. In order to analyze interactions between age and smoking habits it was necessary to acquire nine additional speakers, especially young and elderly smokers.
The speakers were grouped according to their chronological age (young vs. elderly) as well as according to their smoking habits (non-smokers vs. smokers).

Table 1. Descriptive statistics of elderly speakers' age grouped by age category and smoking habits.

SPEAKER GROUP	N	MEAN	SD	MIN	MAX
Young non-smoker	6	26.0	1.79	24	28
Young smoker	6	25.3	1.51	24	28
Elderly non-smoker	6	63.2	4.96	55	68
Elderly smoker	6	59.8	5.35	55	68

In this study *young* refers to young adulthood. The young non-smokers are on average 26.0 years old. The group mean age of the young smokers is 25.3 years. Taking into account the difference of 0.7 years, both groups have a comparable mean age. The attribute *elderly* refers to advanced adulthood. Here the elderly non-smokers are on average 63.2 years, the elderly smokers 59.8 years old (see Table 1). Because each speaker was assigned either to the group of young or to the group of elderly people, which in turn is a quite rough categorisation, the mean difference of 3.4 years between elderly smokers and non-smokers was accepted. It should be noted that the range of the speakers' chronological age is identical for smokers and non-smokers. Assigning a speaker either to the group of smokers or to the group of non-smokers is quite arbitrary. There are no natural rules that could be applied in order to separate speakers into groups of intermittent, or weak, or heavy smokers. In this study, at the beginning of a recording session speakers were asked to give information regarding their smoking habits. According to this information speakers were grouped into smokers and non-smokers afterwards. Similar to the two levels of chronological age the grouping of women into smokers vs. non-smokers is a fairly rough approximation of the smoking habits. Speakers who claimed to smoke ten or more cigarettes per day were considered as smokers. One exception was one elderly woman who claimed to have smoked more or less for 50 years. Because of the rather large number of years she had smoked this woman was considered as smoker too, although she smoked less than 10 cigarettes per day. All speakers participated voluntarily and were not rewarded.

2.2 Recordings

The recordings were produced with high quality audio equipment (microphone AKG C 410 headset or Sennheiser ME 64, DAT TASCAM DA P1 or DAT Sony TCD D 8) in a quiet environment. Most speakers were recorded in a sound protected booth. Some speakers were recorded at their home. In such cases it was ensured that no external sounds interfered with the woman's voice. The audio signals were recorded with a sampling frequency of 44.1 kHz. Prior to the perception test all signals were normalised with respect to their amplitude. Signals were cut at zero crossings to avoid clicks during the listening test.

The full speech material originally comprised sustained vowels, single words, a read short story and spontaneous speech (for details see Winkler, 2009). Results in the literature (Schötz, 2006; Winkler, 2009) have shown that single spoken words already include a huge amount of information to signal a speaker's age. The linguistic structure is simple and therefore single words are appropriate for acoustic analysis and comparability of results. It was decided to use three words per speaker: the German words 'Lawine' (Engl. avalanche),'klimatisieren' (Engl. to air-condition) and 'massiv' (Engl. solid). The words were chosen for the following reasons: The corpus should contain words already used in a previous age estimation task (see Winkler, 2009, p.133) with quite high accuracy for 'klimatisieren' and 'Lawine' as well as rather low accuracy for 'massiv'. The word 'klimatisieren' was included because of its substantial length of five syllables. At the other end of the accuracy, 'massiv' was included because it was the shortest word (two syllables) of the words that performed worse in a previous perception test. The remaining word was chosen because of its high accuracy achieved in a previous test combined with a medium length (three syllables, 'Lawine'). The full speech material used in this study should contain words of different lengths (i.e. number of syllables) and of different recognition accuracy in order to obtain results that are as independent as possible of the exact phonetic content of the respective words. The perception tests contained exactly one production of each word for each speaker. The number of speech items presented to the listeners twice was thus 24 (speakers) x 3 (words) = 72.

2.3 Listener group

A total of twelve listeners, eight females and four males, participated in the perception test. Most listeners were young. The average age (and SD) of the group of female listeners was 26.8 (5.3) years. The male listeners had an average age of 29.8 (6.9) years. All participants reported normal hearing abilities. Previous perception tests containing parts of this speech material (see Winkler, 2009, section 4.3.1) have shown that even averaging over the judgments of only twelve listeners leads to rather accurate average perceived age judgments.

2.4 Perception tests

The perception tests were organized so that judgments of age and smoking habits would be naturally uncorrelated. Specifically, the test was organised in two parts. Every participant rated the age for all 72 stimuli and after finishing the first part she/ he then judged smoking habits. For both parts and each participant the stimuli were presented in random order. Both parts, perceived age and smoking habits, were arranged by the praat perception test environment (Boersma, 2006). All participants used headphones.

Within the context of this study the judgment response time was not considered crucial and thus was not limited. However, listeners were instructed to base their judgment on their first impression. Initially, a participant listened to one speech item. After choosing a response, a 250 ms pause followed before the next item was presented. Each stimulus, if required, could be repeated once.

2.4.1 Determining perceived age

For the judgment of age a test design was applied that does not ask for direct age judgment but for an age range of five years. To rate the age, listeners choose one of 16 boxes labelled with an age value (in years). The box for the youngest possible rating referred to a perceived age of 15, and the box for the oldest possible rating to a perceived age of 90 years. In the graphical user interface for age estimation the boxes were arranged side by side to visually approximate an age continuum.
The mean perceived age per stimulus was derived for further statistical analyses by averaging the judgments of all listeners for a given speech item.

2.4.2 Determining perceived smoking habits

Similar strategies were used to obtain and compile the ratings for the perceived smoking habits. At the beginning it was not clear how accurately listeners would be able to judge smoking habits. It was decided to use four alternative response categories only, with the leftmost category labelled with "zero cigarettes per day" and the rightmost category with "more than 20 cigarettes per day". Before starting the listening test, every listener read an instruction sheet which explained that the first box referred to non-smokers, whereas the rightmost box referred to a heavy smoker. The remaining two boxes were labelled with "less than ten" and "more than ten" cigarettes per day, giving listeners the possibility to rate less extreme gradations. Again, these judgments were averaged per speech item in order to reduce error variance. All computations and statistical analyses were obtained with R (Development Core Team, 2008).

3 Results

3.1 Perceived age

The results of the perception test regarding the average perceived age are depicted in Figure 1. Since perceived age was analyzed with respect to smoking habits, the results are provided for smokers and non-smokers separately.

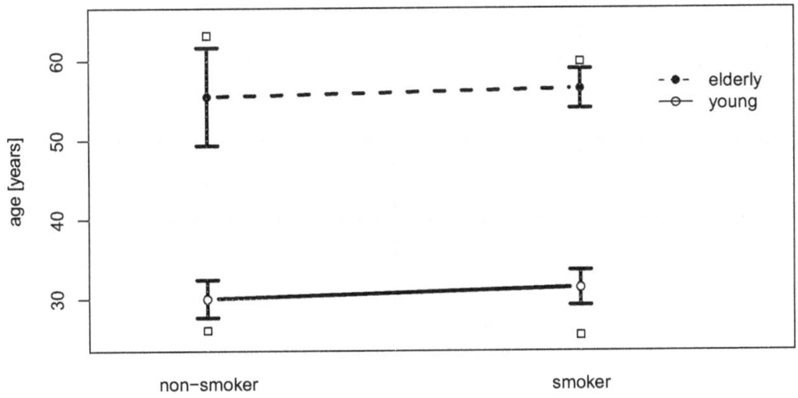

Figure 1. Group means of perceived age values grouped by the smoking habit. Error bars represent 95% CI. Squares represent group means of chronological age.

The group of young non-smokers (average PA = 30.0 years, SD = 4.8 years) was overestimated by an amount of 4.0 years, whereas the group of young smokers (mean PA = 31.4 years, SD = 4.4 years) was judged to be 6.1 years older than their group mean chronological age. The majority of elderly speakers were judged to be younger than their respective chronological age. The amount of underestimation was 7.7 years for the non-smokers (mean PA = 55.5 years, SD = 12.4 years) and 3.4 years for the smokers (mean PA = 56.4 years, SD = 5.0 years).

In order to test which factors influenced the perceived age, a repeated measure ANOVA was applied, with mean perceived age as the dependent variable, chronological age group, the word, and smoking habits as

the independent variables, and a correction for the speaker repetitions. The ANOVA revealed a statistically significant effect for the chronological age group ($F[1,20] = 84.30$, $p < 0.001$). No other effects reached statistical significance.
The amount of overestimation of the age of the young speakers (4.0 and 6.1 years) falls well into the range determined previously (5.4 to 7.7 years in Winkler (2009, p.271)). Underestimation of the age of the elderly is present, but with -7.7 and -3.4 years even smaller than previously obtained (-6.4 to -14.7 years depending on the word, Winkler (see 2009, p.271)).

3.2 Perceived smoking habits

The ratings of smoking habit are not normally distributed because of the rating scale used. Hence ratings of perceived smoking habits are described in terms of median and quartiles. The box plot in Figure 2 shows that the group of young smokers received on the average greater values of smoking habits (median = 0.66) than the group of young non-smokers (median = 0.38). A similar pattern but higher values were determined for the elderly speakers. Judged smoking habits were greater for smokers (median = 2.00) than for non-smokers (median = 1.04). Notches for smokers and non-smokers of comparable age, however, do not overlap, so that a separation of non-smokers and smokers of comparable age seems possible.
In order to quantify these findings, a Wilcoxon rank sum test with continuity correction (one-sided) was applied to the data of young and elderly women separately, with perceived smoking habit as the dependent variable and the smoking habit as the independent variable. The analysis revealed statistically significant differences between scores of smokers and non-smokers for both young ($W=69$, $p<0.01$) and elderly ($W=55$, $p<0.001$) speakers.
This result shows that perceived tobacco consumption is significantly affected by the smoking habit of a speaker if the chronological age group is considered. The boxplots in Figure 2 further show that judgment of smoking habits is strongly influenced by the chronological age of the speaker. This interrelation is investigated within the following section.

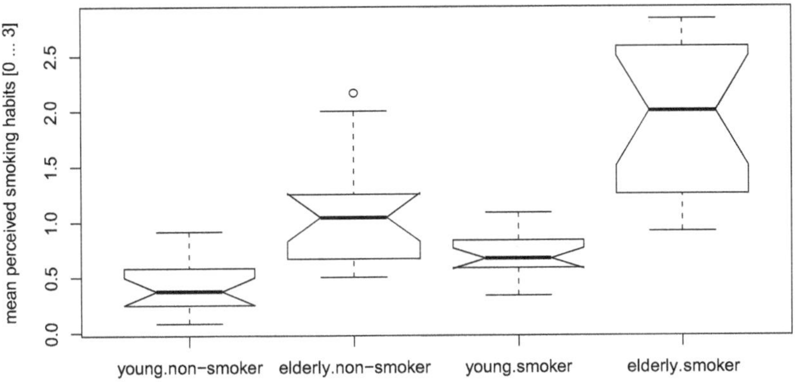

Figure 2. Box plots of the perceived smoking habits based on ratings of words spoken by young and elderly non-smokers (left) and smokers (right). Notches give a rough approximation of the 95% CI for the medians.

3.3 Relation between age estimation and smoking

? Results in section 3.1 have shown that age estimation is not significantly influenced by the smoking habit of a speaker. However, it is noticed in Figure 2 that, independent of the smoking habit, ratings of smoking habits seem to depend on the age of a speaker. The boxplot indicates that judgment of smoking habits rises as the age of a speaker increases. Paradoxically elderly non-smokers achieved greater values than young smokers. In other words, elderly non-smokers were perceived to smoke more cigarettes per day than young smokers.

In order to analyze this observation quantitatively, a Wilcoxon rank sum test with continuity correction (one-sided) was applied with perceived smoking habits as dependent variable and chronological age group as independent variable. The test reveals that ratings for elderly speakers are significantly greater ($W=128.5$, $p<0.001$) than the ratings for young speakers. This means that listeners are significantly influenced by the age of a speaker in judging a speaker's smoking habit. The relation between the mean perceived age and the mean perceived smoking habit is visualized in Figure 3.

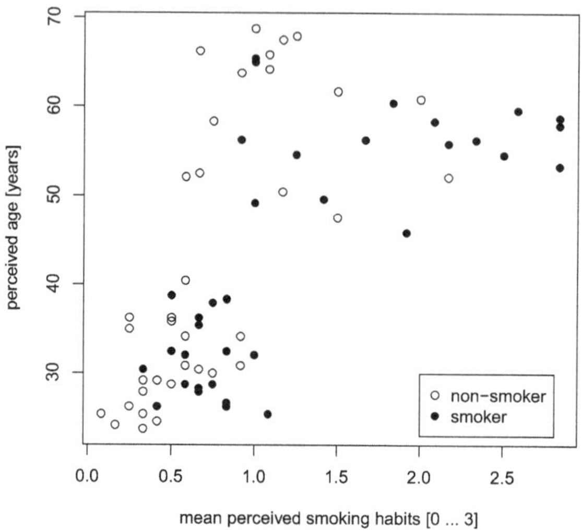

Figure 3. Relation between average perceived age and average perceived smoking habits of words spoken by young and elderly women; data were labelled with regard to the actual smoking habit (see legend).

It shows that listeners predominantly used the first two categories for judging smoking habits of young speakers (lower left quarter in Figure 3), referring to no or very low tobacco consumption. To judge elderly speakers the second and third category, referring to very low and moderate tobacco consumption was used to discriminate between non-smokers and smokers. Data in Figure 3 clearly show a right-shift of the elderly speakers on the 4-point rating scale of perceived smoking habit. The data in Figure 3 further support the results of section 3.1, where age estimations were not significantly influenced by the smoking habits of the speakers. In the scatter plot of perceptual data (Figure 3) it could be observed that comparable actual smoking habits lead to different judgments. The data in Figure 3 do not show strong evidence for increased age estimations caused by heavier perceived smoking habits within the groups of comparable age. The graph contains data of elderly actual non-smokers (unfilled circle) with relatively low perceived smoking habit but remarkable high age estimations.

4 Discussion

The aim of this study was to analyze the possible influence of smoking and perceived smoking habits on age estimations. First it was shown that a group of twelve listeners on the average was able to differentiate between young and elderly speakers. Then it was shown that listeners successfully separated between non-smokers and smokers, at least if the chronological age group of the speaker was taken into account. The main finding of this study is that, while judgment of smoking habit heavily relied on the chronological age of a speaker, age estimations have not been influenced significantly by a speakers' smoking habit. Examples were given for which listeners judged speakers to have only a weak smoking habit but nevertheless an averaged perceived age of about 70 years.

In this study listeners were able to estimate the age of young and elderly speakers with reasonable accuracy. Group mean of chronological age and group mean of perceived age values differ by an amount of -3.4 (smokers) and -7.7 years (non-smokers) in elderly voices. This is comparable to average differences previously reported by Braun (1996) for speakers ranging between 25 and 59 years of age, who used read speech to determine a difference of about -6 years. These results are further in line with differences of -6.4 to -14.7 years reported in Winkler (2009), where the same words but slightly different speakers (all non-smokers) were examined in a comparable perception test design. Regarding the voices of young speakers, the difference between chronological and perceived age of 4.0 (non-smokers) and 6.1 years (smokers) is comparable with values between 5.4 and 7.7 years previously determined by Winkler (2009) and slightly worse than the difference of about three years obtained by Nagao (2006) for young speakers. The slightly more exact result of Nagao could be explained by the fact that she used short phrases, which may contain more acoustic cues than the single words used in this study.

It was not possible to determine the accuracy exactly because of the quantised rating scale used. The voices were rated by choosing an age value representing an age range of five years. The decision to use this kind of scale was based on two assumptions: Firstly, results from literature suggest that a single listener does not achieve accuracies higher than five years. Secondly, it was assumed that ratings are equally distributed around a mean, leading to the measure of the mean perceived age per stimulus by averaging over the ratings of all listeners. However, to avoid downscaling of the chronological age scale to five year differences, in this study age estimations were used directly and were analysed related to the binary age grouping (i.e. young and elderly).

While performance of listeners is well studied in the context of age estimations (Shipp and Hollien, 1969; Ryan and Burk, 1974; Hartman, 1979; Neiman and Applegate, 1990; Braun and Cerrato, 1999), to our knowledge listeners' performance regarding perception of smoking has not been tested before. This may be due to the problem that no natural scale exists to determine speakers' smoking habits. The distinction between smoker and non-smoker might be based on the observation of not smoking at all in contrast to any kind of tobacco consumption. However, consumption of very little tobacco may not lead to perceivable acoustic cues in the voices of the speakers classified as smokers based on the rule given above. Hence, it is hard to define ranges of typical smoking habits. Furthermore, it is questionable to what degree results from different age groups could be compared. An elderly speaker smoking 20 cigarettes per day has probably been smoking a significantly longer length of time than a 20-year-old speaker with comparable smoking habits. Beside the exact smoking habit its duration might have an influence on the acoustic voice characteristics. To take these problems into account, in this study a quite rough categorization was chosen to define the categories "smoker" and "non-smoker" based on the reports of the speakers regarding their smoking habits. The results of the influence of smoking habits on age estimation are discussed for young and elderly women separately.

Results regarding the smoking habits indicate that listeners perform well in judging tobacco consumption of women, if the age group of the speaker is taken into account. The distribution of judgments (see Figure 2) suggests that listeners do not separate speakers into non-smokers and smokers in a binary way. Listeners seem to be quite sensitive in interpreting signs of tobacco consumption. The filled circles in Figure 3 further show the different judgments for all smokers.

Figure 2 displays that elderly non-smokers achieved greater values of smoking habits than the young smokers, indicating that perceived tobacco consumption strongly depends on a speakers' age. Given that for each age group smokers achieved significantly greater values than non-smokers, listeners seem to take into account the age of a speaker in judging smoking habits. The scatter plot in Figure 3 clearly shows that elderly speakers were judged, on the average, to have higher tobacco consumption. The scatter plot further shows that the range the listeners use to judge smoking habits is smaller for young than for elderly women. At first glance it seems that young smokers do not show strong enough acoustic cues to be judged to have heavy smoking habits. This might be related to the relative short duration they smoke. On the other hand this could not explain the observation that no elderly non-smoker achieved an average perceived smoking habit in the region of the perceptual category "non-smoker".

Given that listeners' judgments rely on acoustic features of the speech signal, it follows that speech signals of young speakers and the elderly contain acoustic cues signalling age and smoking habits to some extent separately. While age estimations were rather stable, the age clearly influences the perceived smoking habits. These results could be interpreted as follows: There is a rather complex pattern of acoustic cues evaluated by listeners to estimate a speakers' age. Another set of acoustic cues, primarily comprising mean fundamental frequency and voice quality parameters, give hints on the tobacco consumption. It is further assumed that there is a subset of acoustic features that signal age as well as smoking habits. In addition to these "shared" subset features, other characteristics, for instance tempo information or prosodic cues may signal primarily age, which would explain the comparatively stable age estimations. On the contrary, lack of additional characteristics besides the "shared" subset of acoustic features may explain the strong influence of age on perceived smoking habits.

This interpretation could explain why elderly speakers, who usually show degradation of voice to some extent, always get higher judgments of their smoking habits. It would further explain why young smokers, although showing signs of voice degradation necessary for successful judgment of smoking habit, do not achieve higher age estimations. Although the laryngeal function may decline caused by increased tobacco consumption, there are probably enough additional features indicating that the speaker is quite young.

In Braun (1996) listeners judged, on the average, smokers to be 3.0 years (expert listener) or 2.7 years (student listener) older than their group mean of chronological age. Contrarily, non-smokers of comparable age were judged to be 1.9 years (experts) or 3.1 years (student listener) younger. From these observations it was concluded that heavy smoking habit increases the perceived age. Although distribution of the chronological age of the speakers differs remarkably, this effect was observed in this study as well (see Figure 1). This effect, however, did not reach statistical significance in this study. It could be considered as a bias that is weak in amplitude but usually present for smokers because of indices of a declined laryngeal function.
The even smaller influence of smoking on age estimation in this study (1.3 years for smokers, -1.9 years for non-smokers) may be explained by a tendency of listeners to underestimate the age of the elderly, and to overestimate the age of young speakers (centralisation effect). The demonstration of the influence of smoking on age estimation in Braun (1996) was based on speakers whose age ranged between 25 and 59 years. In this study, however, where only young (24-28 years) and elderly speakers (55-68 years) participated, all speakers were strongly influenced by the centralisation effect. As a conclusion one may say, that the influence of smoking on age estimations may appear slightly stronger in the voices of speakers in the middle of adulthood, and may even decrease in the voices of very young and elderly speakers because of the influence of the centralisation effect.
Interestingly, in the study of Braun (1996) experts as well as student listeners were more accurate in estimating the correct age of the smokers than that of the non-smokers. In this study, although accuracy was not determined explicitly, data in Figure 1 suggest that for young speakers listeners' accuracy is higher for non-smokers, but it is higher for elderly smokers than for elderly non-smokers. This pattern could directly result from the interrelation between influences of age and the centralisation effect. Because of the overestimation of young speakers and a positive bias caused by recognition of smoking habits, age estimation for young smokers would further increase and, hence, accuracy would decrease. In the case of elderly smokers, whose age is underestimated because of the centralisation effect, the positive bias induced by recognition of smoking habit would counteract centralisation and,

hence, would increase the resulting age estimation accuracy. In summary, it could be speculated that accuracy of age estimation is higher for non-smokers in young adulthood as well as for smokers in advanced adulthood.
While Braun (1996) used read speech to demonstrate the effect of smoking habits on perceived age, the speech material used in the present study was rather short. Our results show that single words comprised of only two syllables allow for fairly good judgments of a speaker's smoking habit and age. Single words are phonetically less complex than read speech. Since a judgment of smoking habits and age is possible even in case of single words, this kind of speech material could be used to identify the acoustic features that exclusively and simultaneously signal age and smoking habits within successive studies.

5 Acknowledgements

Support in the acquisition and recordings of elderly smoking women was provided by Susanne Fuchs. Furthermore I gratefully acknowledge the comments and very helpful suggestions of Laura Koenig, Pascal Perrier and another reviewer on an earlier version of the manuscript.

References

Baken, R. (2005). The aged voice: A new hypothesis. *Journal of Voice*, 19(3):317–325.

Boersma, P. & Weenink, D. (2006). Praat: Doing phonetics by computer (version 4.5.01). [computer program].

Braun, A. (1996). Age estimation by different listener groups. *Forensic Linguistics*, 3 (1):65–73.

Braun, A. and Cerrato, L. (1999). Estimating speaker age across languages. In *Proceedings of the International Congress of Phonetic Sciences, San Francisco*, volume 99, pages 1369–1372.

Brückl, M. and Sendlmeier, W. (2003). Aging female voices: An acoustic and perceptive analysis. In *Proceedings of the ISCA Workshop Voice Quality: Functions, Analysis and Synthesis (VOQUAL)*, page 163–168. ISCA.

de Pinto, O. and Hollien, H. (1982). Speaking fundamental frequency characteristics of Australian women: Then and now. *Journal of Phonetics*, 10:367–375.

Decoster, W. and Debruyne, F. (2000). Longitudinal voice changes: facts and interpretation. *Journal of Voice*, 14(2):184–193.

Development Core Team, R. (2008). *R: A language and environment for statistical computing. R Foundation for Statistical Computing.*

Gilbert, H. and Weismer, G. (1974). The effects of smoking on the speaking fundamental frequency of adult women. *Journal of Psycholinguistic Research*, 3(3):225–231.

Harnsberger, J., Shrivastav, R., Brown, W., Rothman, H., and Hollien, H. (2006). Speaking rate and fundamental frequency as speech cues to perceived age. *Journal of Voice*, 22(1):58–69.

Harrington, J., Palethorpe, S., and Watson, C. (2007). Age-related changes in fundamental frequency and formants: A longitudinal study of four speakers. In *Proceedings of Interspeech*, page 2753–2756.

Hartman, D. (1979). The perceptual identity and characteristics of aging in normal male adult speakers. *Journal of Communication Disorders*, 12(1):53–61.

Hecker, M. and Kreul, E. (1971). Descriptions of the speech of patients with cancer of the vocal folds. Part I: Measures of fundamental frequency. *The Journal of the Acoustical Society of America*, 49:1275–1289.

Hollien, H. and Tolhurst, G. (1978). The Aging Voice. In Weinberg, G., editor, *Transcripts of the Seventh Symposium on Care of the Professional Voice, Volume II: Life Span Changes in the Human Voice*, page 67–73. The Voice Foundation.

Honjo, I. and Isshiki, N. (1980). Laryngoscopic and voice characteristics of aged persons. *Archives of Otolaryngology*, 106(3):149–150.

Huntley, R., Hollien, H., and Shipp, T. (1987). Influences of listener characteristics on perceived age estimations. *Journal of Voice*, 1(1):49–52.

Jacques, R. and Rastatter, M. (1990). Recognition of speaker age from selected acoustic features as perceived by normal young and older listeners. *Folia Phoniatrica*, 42(3):118–124.

Kreul, E. and Hecker, M. (1971). Description of the speech of patients with cancer of the vocal folds. Part II: Judgments of age and voice quality. *Journal of the Acoustical Society of America*, 49:1283–1287.

Linville, S. (1987). Acoustic-perceptual studies of aging voice in women. *Journal of Voice*, 1(1):44–48.

Linville, S. (1996). The sound of senescence. *Journal of Voice*, 10(2):190–200.

Linville, S. (2001). *Vocal Aging.* Singular Thomson Learning, San Diego.

Linville, S. and Fisher, H. (1985). Acoustic characteristics of perceived versus actual vocal age in controlled phonation by adult females. *Journal of the Acoustical Society of America*, 78(1):40–48.

Linville, S. and Korabic, E. (1986). Elderly listeners' estimates of vocal age in adult females. *The Journal of the Acoustical Society of America*, 80:692–694.

Mueller, P. (1997). The Aging Voice. In *Seminars in Speech and Language*, volume 18, pages 159–170. Thieme Medical Publishers Inc.

Nagao, K. (2006). *Cross-language study of age perception.* PhD thesis, Indiana University.

Neiman, G. and Applegate, J. (1990). Accuracy of listener judgments of perceived age relative to chronological age in adults. *Folia Phoniatrica*, 42(6):327–330.

Nishio, M. and Niimi, S. (2008). Changes in speaking fundamental frequency characteristics with aging. *Folia Phoniatrica et Logopaedica*, 60(3):120–127.

Orlikoff, R. (1990). The relationship of age and cardiovascular health to certain acoustic characteristics of male voices. *Journal of Speech, Language and Hearing Research*, 33:450–457.

Orlikoff, R. and Baken, R. (1990). Consideration of the relationship between the fundamental frequency of phonation and vocal jitter. *Folia Phoniatrica*, 42(1):31–40.

Ptacek, P. and Sander, E. (1966). Age recognition from voice. *Journal of Speech and Hearing Research*, 9(2):273–277.

Ryan, W. and Burk, K. (1974). Perceptual and acoustic correlates of aging in the speech of males. *Journal of Communication Disorders*, 7(2):181–192.

Schötz, S. (2005). Effects of stimulus duration and type on perception of female and male speaker age. In *Proceedings of FONETIK*, page 87–90.

Schötz, S. (2006). *Perception, Analysis and Synthesis of Speaker Age.* PhD thesis, Lund University.

Shipp, T. and Hollien, H. (1969). Perception of the aging male voice. *Journal of Speech, Language and Hearing Research*, 12(4):704–710.

Shipp, T., Qi, Y., Huntley, R., and Hollien, H. (1992). Acoustic and temporal correlates of perceived age. *Journal of Voice*, 6(3):211–216.

Shrivastav, R., Hollien, H., Brown, W., Rothman, H., and Harnsberger, J. (2003). Shifting Perceptions of Age in Voice. In *poster, 146th Meeting of the Acoustical Society of America.*

Stölten, K. and Engstrand, O. (2002). Effects of sex and age in the Arjeplog dialect: A listening test and measurements of preaspiration and VOT. *TMH-QPSR*, 44:29–32.

Stoicheff, M. (1981). Speaking fundamental frequency characteristics of nonsmoking female adults. *Journal of Speech and Hearing Research*, 24(3):437–441.

Verdonck-de Leeuw, I. and Mahieu, H. (2004). Vocal aging and the impact on daily life: A longitudinal study. *Journal of Voice*, 18(2):193–202.

Winkler, R. (2007a). Influences of pitch and speech rate on the perception of age from voice. In *Proceedings of the International Congress of Phonetic Sciences, Saarbrücken*, pages 1849–1852.

Winkler, R. (2007b). Testing the relevance of speech rate, pitch and a glottal chink for the perception of age in synthesized speech using formant synthesis. In *Proceedings of Interspeech*, pages 2653–2656.

Winkler, R. (2009). *Merkmale junger und alter Stimmen: Analyse ausgewählter Parameter im Kontext von Wahrnehmung und Klassifikation*. PhD thesis, Logos Verlag, Berlin.

Winkler, R. and Sendlmeier, W. (2006). EGG open quotient in aging voices-changes with increasing chronological age and its perception. *Logopedics Phonatrics Vocology*, 31(2):51–56.

Xue, S. and Deliyski, D. (2001). Effects of aging on selected acoustic voice parameters: Preliminary normative data and educational implications. *Educational Gerontology*, 27(2):159–168.

Modeling Different Voice Qualities for Female and Male Talkers Using a Geometric-Kinematic Articulatory Voice Source Model: Preliminary Results

BERND J. KRÖGER*
PETER BIRKHOLZ
JIM KANNAMPUZHA
CHRISTIANE NEUSCHAEFER-RUBE

Abstract: Modeling natural sounding voice qualities – for example the pressed-modal-breathy voice quality continuum which widely occurs during normal speech production – is a crucial point in speech synthesis. A parametric voice source model using prescribed sinusoidal vocal fold vibration patterns (i.e. extended Titze model) is introduced in this paper. This voice source model was adapted for synthesis of a typical male and female voice. A simulation experiment was performed by varying glottal abduction/adduction in order to generate a voice quality continuum from pressed over modal towards breathy. A parameter analysis of the resulting waveshapes of glottal flow and its time derivative was carried out in terms of the LF-model. This analysis indicates that our parametric voice source model is flexible enough to generate the modal to breathy but not the modal to pressed voice quality continuum for the male as well as for the female voice. It can be hypothesized that a self-oscillating voice source

* This paper is dedicated to the 60th Birthday of Bernd Pompino-Marschall. I met Bernd Pompino-Marschall in the early 90th of the last century as a young scientist when Bernd already was Professor in Berlin. I thank him especially for supporting me in my hard years between PhD and getting my permanent position at RWTH Aachen University. In these years I always was welcome to visit his Lab at ZAS and at Humboldt University of Berlin and I was employed in Berlin from 1999 to 2000. Great times! I learned a lot! Thank you for all, Bernd!

model is needed in order to generate the whole spectrum of vocal fold vibration patterns occurring during normal speech production.

1 Introduction

The problem of generating natural sounding voices as well as generating changes in voice quality is not yet solved for parametric voice source models used in articulation-based speech synthesis systems. Since natural voice quality is a key for reaching high quality synthetic speech, corpus-based synthesis is currently used if high quality speech is needed (Clark et al., 2007). But changes in voice quality as they occur during the production of utterances (e.g. normal to pressed and normal to breathy, Klatt and Klatt (1990) as well as differences in voice quality due to different speaking styles or due to different emotional states of speakers cannot be realized easily in corpus-based approaches. In addition, if the synthesis of different voices is demanded (e.g. male vs. female or child vs. adult), corpus-based systems need one complete speech corpus for each voice. Furthermore, modeling huge differences in loudness as well as modeling huge differences in pitch is not unproblematic if corpus-based speech synthesis is used. Thus, if a variety of natural sounding voice qualities is demanded, i.e. different speakers, different voice qualities, huge loudness and pitch ranges, it would be advantageous to use other approaches, e.g. articulation-based or comparable parametric speech synthesis approaches. But currently the segmental as well as prosodic quality of these systems is not as high as that of corpus-based approaches.
The quality of articulation-based speech synthesis increased dramatically over the last decades. Huge corpora of kinematic data (EMA, EPG, MRI) are now available for developing realistic models for vocal tract geometries of speech sounds as well as for developing approaches for modeling coarticulation and vocal tract kinematics (Badin et al., 2002; Engwall, 2003; Birkholz and Kröger, 2006; Serrurier and Badin, 2008). In addition, the knowledge concerning vocal tract acoustics and aerodynamics increased (see the overview on vocal tract acoustics given by Stevens, 1998), which now allows the development of high quality articulatory-acoustic models (e.g. Birkholz et al., 2007). Furthermore a lot of knowledge is currently available concerning the voice source and

its integration in articulation-based synthesis systems (e.g. Titze, 1989a; Story and Titze, 1995; Titze and Story, 2002).

Breathy voice quality, modal (or normal) voice quality, and pressed voice quality (sometimes used synonymously with the terms creaky or laryngealized) can occur within the realization of a single utterance (Klatt and Klatt, 1990). Thus these qualities can be seen as phonation subtypes occurring during speech, i.e. during the use of the chest register as basic phonation type. The change from modal to breathy voice quality occurs within sentence production, for example by changing from a normal or stressed to an unstressed syllable (Gobl and Chasaide, 1988). A change from normal to pressed voice quality often occurs at the end of an utterance in order to signalize finality (Klatt and Klatt, 1990). In this paper we will not focus on creak or laryngealization but on breathy, modal, and pressed. The voice qualities breathy and pressed can easily be reached from modal voice quality at nearly all pitch levels within the chest register - i.e. without any "register break ", (see Sundberg, 1987, p. 50 for the definition of the term "register break ") - while creaky voice, laryngealized voice, as well as breathy-laryngealized voice only occur at very low pitches (Klatt and Klatt, 1990) and thus should be treated as phonation types occurring within a separate voice register - i.e. vocal fry or pulse register, (see Sundberg, 1987, p. 50) for the definition of these registers - or at least as special types of vocal fold vibration occurring at the lower edge of the chest register.

The pressed-modal-breathy voice quality continuum is realized by varying mainly one physiological voice source control parameter, i.e. *glottal or vocal fold abduction/adduction.* (i) During glottal abduction vocal folds become more and more separated from each other by an outward translation or rotation of the arytenoid cartilages, but this separation is not sufficiently large to cause vocal fold vibration to cease. This abduction process changes voice quality from modal to breathy. (ii) After glottal adduction, vocal folds are (softly) adducted. A further increasing adduction results in medial compression that activates a force which occurs perpendicular to the length of the vocal folds on the level of the vocal processes and modal voice quality now changes towards pressed voice quality.

A lot of evidence exists for the fact that two dimensions of control are sufficient in order to describe phonemic contrasts produced by the voice source as well as the phonetic variability of the voice source during normal (i.e. emotionally neutral) utterance production. (i) Firstly, changes in fundamental frequency (F0) lead to distinctive contrast in many languages (i.e. tone languages). In addition, changes in F0 occur within all languages as a phonetic realization feature for intonation and thus for prosody. Physiologically, changes in F0 mainly result from varying *vocal fold tension* which occurs parallel to the length of the vocal folds. (ii) Secondly, changes in voice quality with respect to breathy vs. modal vs. pressed occur as a phonemic contrast in some languages (Klatt and Klatt, 1990; Gordon and Ladefoged, 2001). In addition, these changes in voice quality occur within many languages as a phonetic feature of stress as well as sentence or utterance finality (see above). Furthermore, vocal fold or glottal abduction is the main control dimension for the linguistically important voiced-voiceless sound contrast while glottal adduction in addition is the main control dimension for the voiced sound to glottal stop contrast: If abduction is stronger than for changing voice quality from normal to breathy, vocal fold vibration ends and voicelessness occurs; if adduction is stronger than for changing voice quality from normal to pressed, vocal vibration ends as well and a glottal stop is produced.

Voice source models should reflect these facts by introducing *two main voice source control parameters*, i.e. (i) vocal fold tension resulting from forces occurring parallel to the length of the vocal folds and (ii) glottal abduction/adduction including medial compression resulting from forces perpendicular to the length of the vocal folds on the level of the vocal processes. On the basis of this control paradigm, voice source models should be able (i) to produce F0 variation, (ii) to produce the voiceless to voiced sound to glottal stop contrast, and (iii) to produce the typical vocal fold vibration patterns and the typical acoustic features of the voice quality continuum breathy-modal-pressed.

The physiological differences of the male vs. female voice source as well as the resulting glottal flow waveshapes and acoustic features are described in the literature (e.g. Holmberg et al., 1988; Titze, 1989c; Hanson and Chuang, 1999; Karlsson, 1992; Karlsson and Liljencrants, 1996). These settings and features are listed in detail in section 2 of this paper as a basis for our modeling experiment (section 4). It should be noted that female voices in general are found to be more breathy than male voices,

which makes it interesting to model male vs. female voice quality together with modeling the pressed-modal-breathy voice quality continuum. The physiological or voice source settings as well as the resulting glottal flow waveshapes and acoustic features for breathy, modal, and pressed voice quality for both male and female speakers are described in the literature, e.g.Klatt and Klatt (1990), Karlsson and Liljencrants (1996) and these settings and features are listed in section 3 of this paper as a further basis of our modeling experiment.
The articulation-based speech synthesis system used for our simulation experiment is a geometric-kinematic model. No detailed neuromuscular and no detailed biomechanical modeling of the vocal tract articulators (i.e. tongue, lips, lower jaw, velum, larynx) or of the voice source is aimed for in our model. Our vocal tract model comprises a *geometric articulator model* (Birkholz et al., 2006; Birkholz and Kröger, 2006)) driven by a *kinematic articulatory control model* via a set of phonetically motivated *articulatory control parameters* (Kröger and Birkholz, 2007). Our voice source model comprises a *geometric voice source model* as introduced by Titze (1984, 1989a) representing the membranous part of the glottis extended by a permanent bypass for airflow representing the cartilaginous part of the glottis (Kröger, 1997, 1998; Birkholz, 2005). Both parts of the voice source model are driven by a *kinematic voice source control model* via a set of phonetically (i.e. acoustically and articulatorily) motivated *voice source control parameters* (introduced below). In addition the *pulmonary control parameter* lung pressure p_l is introduced. A lung pressure value above phonation threshold pressure (Titze, 1988; Chan and Titze, 2006) is needed for the initiation and maintenance of vocal fold vibration.
While the vocal tract model and its control has already been described in earlier publications (see above), the geometric voice source model and its control is described in detail in section 2 of this paper. In addition the (time invariant) parameterization of the voice source model for a typical male and for a typical female speaker is given. Furthermore a set of (time variant) voice source control parameters capable of adjusting the larynx for the realization of different voice qualities for a male as well as for a female speaker is introduced.

2 The voice source control model

2.1 Structure of the voice source model and its parameters

In our modeling approach, voice source *static* parameters are speaker-specific and time-invariant, i.e. voice source static parameters are capable of adjusting the voice source model with respect to a specific speaker's voice source geometry, while time-variant voice source *dynamic control* parameters specify phonatory gestures generating speech sounds and speech prosody. The set of voice source static parameters directly results from the design of the membranous and cartilaginous part of the voice source model while the set of voice source dynamic control parameters are designed mainly with respect to phonetic criteria for controlling vocal fold activity during speech. It is the task of these dynamic control parameters (i) to generate all segmental voiceless-voiced and voiced-voiceless transitions (i.e. glottal adduction and glottal abduction gestures), (ii) to generate different degrees of stress (sentence stress pattern), intonation contours (sentence intonation pattern), and different loudness levels (soft-normal-loud), and (iii) to generate different voice qualities. The time course of voice source control parameters is generated by the voice source control model.
The *speaker-specific voice source static parameters* for adjusting the voice source with respect to a specific speaker are (i) the *effective length of the membranous and cartilaginous part of the glottis* L_m and L_c and (ii) the *thickness of the glottal constriction* T. It should be emphasized that "effective length" means not "real length" of the vocal folds as occurs if the vocal folds are not vibrating. The effective length of the vocal folds is the midsagittal length of the glottis during vibration (see Figure 1). This effective length is shorter than the real length of the vocal folds, because the vocal folds are bent during vibration (Hollien and Moore, 1960; Titze, 1989c). The real length of the vocal folds is approximately 16 mm for a male and 10 mm for a female speaker. Within the chest register (which is most important for speech) the effective length of the membranous part L_m is different for males and females (as well as the real length) but in addition the effective length varies with frequency. Length values for L_m as estimated after Hollien (1960); Hollien and Moore (1960);

Titze (1989c) for a male and a female voice source and are subsumed in a formula given by Titze (1989a, p.195) for a typical male voice. It can be assumed that the length of the membranous part is shorter by a scale factor of $1/1.6 = 0.625$ for female voices (Titze, 1989c, p.1700). The resulting length values are listed in Table 1.

Table 1. Effective length of membranous part of the glottis L_m and thickness of glottal constriction T as function of fundamental frequency F0 for a standard male and a standard female speaker for the chest register. Estimation after a formula given by Titze (1989b) for the male voice and by using a male to female scaling factor of 0.625 (Titze, 1989c).

MALE VOICE	low	mid-low	mid	mid-high	high
F0 [Hz]	70	90	120	160	200
L_m [mm]	6.2	7.6	8.0	10.2	11.5
T [mm]	11.5	9.5	9.0	7.5	6.3
FEMALE VOICE	low	mid-low	mid	mid-high	high
F0 [Hz]	120	150	200	270	350
L_m [mm]	5.0	6.4	7.2	8.3	9.4
T [mm]	5.6	4.7	3.9	3.4	3.0

The length of the cartilaginous part of the glottis L_c can be estimated as 3 mm for male and 2.5 mm for female speakers (Hirano, 1983; Titze, 1989c). Thickness of the glottal constriction T is different for males and females as well and also depends on frequency (Hollien, 1960; Titze, 1989c). Thickness values for T as estimated after Hollien (1960) and Titze (1989c) are also subsumed in a formula (Titze, 1989a, p.195) and given in Table 1 for the whole range of the chest register (low, mid-low, mid, mid-high, high) for a typical male and female voice. Differences in length and thickness between the male and female voice source can be scaled by the anatomy related scale factor $1/1.2 = 0.83$ for the cartilaginous part of the glottis (Titze, 1989a). It should be noted that the lower scale factor of 0.625 for the membranous part of the glottis (see above) indicates that the vocal folds are a gender-specific human organ.
From the phonetic viewpoint it is advantageous to control the voice source by using two main *voice source dynamic control parameters*, i.e. *vocal fold tension* and *glottal aperture* (i.e. degree of *glottal ab-/adduction*) (see section 1 of this paper). Thus, two different types of *voice source gestures*

or phonatory control gestures are mainly used in articulation-based speech synthesis systems, i.e.(i) *vocal fold tension gestures* and (ii) *glottal abduction and adduction gestures* (see Gordon and Ladefoged, 2001; Kröger, 1993; Kröger, 1998; Kröger and Birkholz, 2007). In order to identify vocal fold tension and glottal aperture in terms of our voice source model it is now necessary to describe our voice source model in more detail. The voice source model of the membranous and cartilaginous part of the glottis is given in Figure 1 (see also Titze, 1984, 1989a; Kröger, 1997; Birkholz, 2005). We can directly identify (i) *effective length of the glottis for the membranous part* L_m and *effective length of the glottis for the cartilaginous part* L_c, (ii) *thickness of the glottal constriction* T, (iii) *cross-sectional area of the glottis for the membranous part* (in the case of vocal fold rest position, also called pre-phonatory state) A_m and for the *cartilaginous part* A_c, (iv) *displacement of posterior membranous part of (symmetrically positioned) vocal folds in rest position* x_m (i.e. displacement of vocal processes, sometimes also called degree of glottal ab-/adduction) and *displacement of the arytenoid cartilages* x_c, (v) *displacement of upper* (or superior) posterior part and *of lower* (or inferior) *posterior membranous part of vocal folds* x_{mu} and x_{ml} with $x_m = (x_{mu} + x_{ml}) * 0.5$ as *mean displacement of the posterior membranous part of the vocal folds* and with $x_{md} = x_{ml} - x_{mu}$ as difference between displacement of upper and lower posterior membranous part of the vocal folds. x_{md} is called *converging rest-position displacement*; $x_{md} > 0$ means: converging vertical glottal shape in rest position as is given in Figure 1b; $x_{md} < 0$ means: diverging vertical glottal shape in rest position. [1] In the case of vocal fold vibration additional parameters need to be introduced. The model can be controlled directly by (i) *fundamental frequency* F0 (i.e. frequency of vocal fold vibration), (ii) *amplitude of vocal fold vibration* x_v (which is equal for the upper and lower part of the vocal folds in this model), and (iii) *phase difference between upper and lower part of vocal*

1 Please notice that all $x_{m...}$-parameters represent displacements or differences of displacements at the (posterior) *end* of the membranous part of the glottis (because the cross-sectional area of this part has a triangular form, Figure 1a), while m_c represents the displacement in the *middle* of the cartilaginous part of the glottis since the cross-sectional area of this part has a trapezoidal form (Figure 1a). Thus, the relationship between cross-sectional glottal area and vocal fold or cartilage *displacement* (which is half of the vocal fold or cartilage *distance*) is $A_c = 2 * x_c * L_c$ for the cartilaginous part and is $A_m = x_m * L_m$ for the membranous part of the glottis (in rest position or pre-phonatory state).

(a)

(b)

(c)

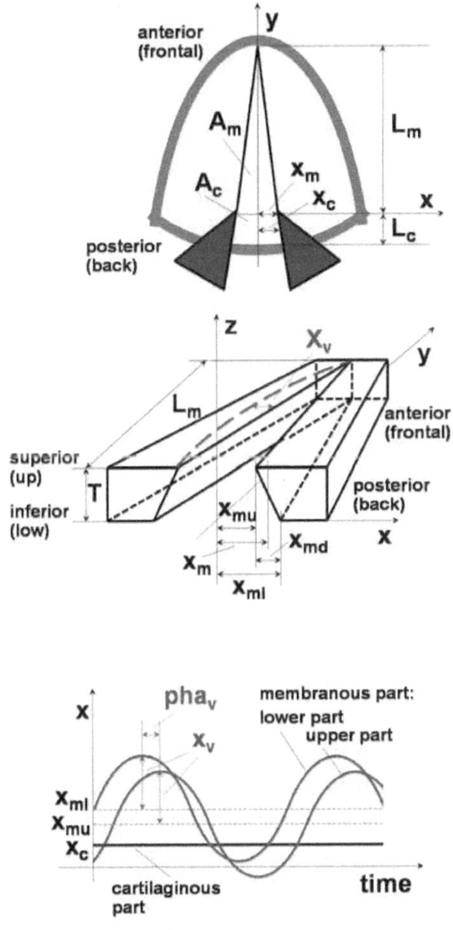

Figure 1. The geometric voice source model. a) View of the vocal folds from above (or horizontal section through the larynx), visualizing the membranous as well as the cartilaginous part of the vocal folds. The filled triangles represent the arytenoid cartilages, the anterior grey arc represents the thyroid cartilage, and the posterior grey arc represents the posterior part of the cricoid cartilage. b) Schematic view of the vocal folds, i.e. of the membranous part of the glottis and its parameterization (after Titze 1984). c) Displacement over time of the upper and lower membranous part of the vocal folds relative to its its rest positions x_{ml} and x_{mu} (dashed lines) during vocal fold vibration. The displacement of the arytenoids cartilages x_c over time is indicated by a black bold line. Vibration patterns in space b) and in time c) are indicated as grey lines. Vibration pattern in space in b) is indicated only for the upper edge of the left vocal fold.

folds pha_v. Some additional remarks concerning our voice source model should be given here: (i) x_m and x_{md} are directly controlled in our voice source model. Thus x_{mu} and x_{ml} are calculated as $x_{mu} = x_m + x_{md} * 0.5$ and $x_{ml} = x_m - x_{md} * 0.5$ (see Figure 1b). (ii) Positive values of x_m directly quantify the degree of abduction for the membranous part of the vocal folds. Negative values for x_m are possible and quantify the degree of adduction and thus quantify the *degree of medial compression* on the vocal folds. This is important if a glottal stop or if pressed voice qualities are modeled.

The vocal fold vibration amplitude x_v is controlled (or calculated) indirectly, depending on the rest position displacement of the membranous part of the glottis x_m and on subglottal pressure p_s (i.e. $x_v = f(x_m, p_s)$ where $p_s = p_l$ in our voice source model) (see Birkholz, 2005, p.40). Vocal fold vibration amplitude x_v increases proportional to p_s^2 (see Titze, 1989b, p.104) and (Birkholz, 2005, p.40) and decreases with increasing glottal ab-/adduction, which leads to an absence of vocal fold vibration if the degree of vocal fold abduction is high (as is needed for example for the realization of voiceless sounds). Other influences on vocal fold vibration amplitude x_v are neglected in this preliminary version of the voice source model.

Now the *voice source dynamic control parameters* vocal fold tension and glottal ab-/adduction can be quantified in terms of our voice source model. (i) It is assumed that vocal fold tension mainly influences fundamental frequency F0 and thus F0 is taken directly as voice source control parameter instead of vocal fold tension. But it should be kept in mind that F0 can be seen here as a direct equivalent to vocal fold tension since in our model F0 has a direct influence on effective length and thickness of the vocal folds (Table 1). (ii) The voice source control parameter *glottal abduction and/or glottal adduction* is quantified by at least four voice source parameters, i.e. displacement of membranous and cartilaginous part of the glottis x_m and x_c, converging rest position displacement x_d, and phase difference of lower versus upper edge of the vocal folds pha_v. The later two parameters (converging rest position displacement and phase difference of lower vs. upper part of the vocal folds) are held constant during glottal ab- and adduction gestures (see below) but the distances of the membranous part and of the cartilaginous part of the glottis x_m and x_c may vary independent from each other even within a single abduction or adduction gesture. This results from different types of movements which can occur for the arytenoids, i.e. rotation and translation. Both types of movements can be superimposed in a single abduction or adduction gesture. Figure 2 illustrates that (i) translation leads to comparable change in x_m and x_c while (ii) rotation mainly leads to changes in x_m while x_c remains constant.

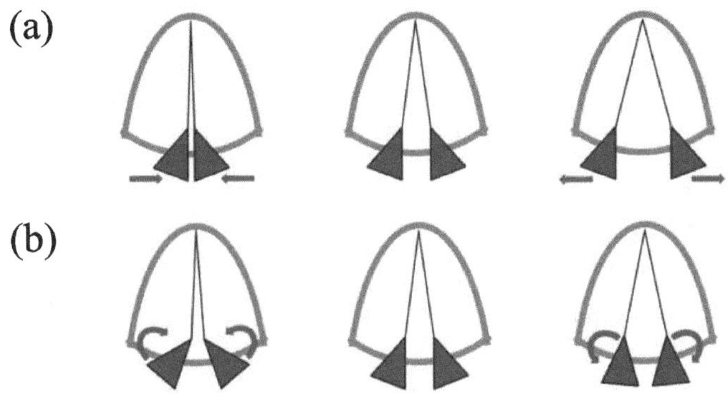

Figure 2. (a) Inward and outward translation. (b) Inward and outward rotation of the arytenoid cartilages occurring in glottal abduction gestures.

2.2 Gestures for controlling voice source activity during speech

While F0 gestures can easily be generated for example by using the Fujisaki approach (Birkholz, 2005, p.111), the situation is more complex for the positioning of the membranous and the cartilaginous part of the glottis for phonation or for segmental voiceless-voiced and voiced-voiceless changes. This laryngeal positioning is realized by glottal abduction and glottal adduction gestures (see Figure 3).

A prominent example for a glottal adduction gesture is the transition of the glottal opening from breathing or from a voiceless sound towards modal phonation. This gesture starts with a wide opening of the glottis where no vocal vibration occurs. The gesture ends with a closure of the glottis (x_m and x_c near 0) and a typical converging vertical shape of the glottis ($x_d > 0$). The best or most effective parameter set for modal

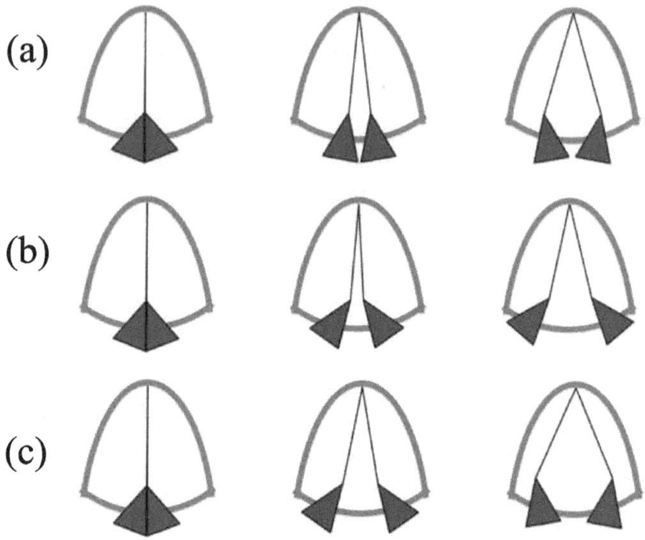

Figure 3. Three abduction gestures with different contributions of outward translation, inward rotation, and outward rotation. Resulting net cross-sectional increase (i.e. resulting overall degree of abduction) is comparable for gestures (a) and (b) but x_m is always smaller during abduction gesture (b) which means, that vocal fold vibration ends at higher values for glottal aperture in this gesture in comparison with gesture (a). Thus gesture (b) is used in our approach for modeling smooth voiced-voiceless transitions and voiceless-voiced transitions. If a higher degree of glottal aperture is needed as can be reached in gesture (b) (e.g. for breathing), a further outward rotation of the arytenoids may occur at high degrees of glottal aperture (c).

phonation can be found by trial and error phonation during modeling voice and speech acquisition (i.e. early phonation stage Kröger et al., 2009). If normal phonation is maintained during the whole utterance the parameters x_d and pha_v can be maintained even during within-sentence abduction-adduction gestures needed for the realization of voiceless segments. In addition for a natural sounding segmental voiceless-voiced transition it is important that vocal fold vibration already starts *before* the adduction gesture has reached its target, i.e. the glottal closure for effective modal phonation. Thus glottal abduction gestures should be able to generate smooth voice onsets and voice offsets (Gobl and Chasaide, 1988). Consequently, the vibrational amplitude x_v of the vocal folds needs to be carefully controlled within glottal abduction gestures.

Since x_v (beside p_l) mainly depends on x_m in our voice source model, a carefully designed control of x_m (together with x_c) is needed. For smooth voice onsets and voice offsets this leads to a translational movement combined with an inward rotational movement of the arytenoid cartilages during voiceless-voiced adduction (Figure 2) as well as vice versa for voiced-voiceless abduction gestures in order to keep x_m small even for medium degrees of abduction (Birkholz, 2005, p. 40).[2]

2.3 Acoustic relevance of voice source parameters

Following the description of our voice source model (see 2.1), six voice source parameters (L_m, L_c,T, x_m, x_c, x_d) describe the geometry of the vocal folds in its rest position (pre-phonatory state) while three parameters (F0, x_v and pha_v) describe vocal fold vibration. A shortcoming of this parameterization is that the waveshape of the cross-sectional glottal area and of the glottal volume flow, which results from vocal fold vibration, cannot be estimated directly. But especially the waveshape of glottal volume flow and of its first time derivative directly reflects important acoustic features of the voice source signal and thus of voice quality (Klatt and Klatt, 1990). Thus we will introduce now a parameterization of the waveshape of glottal flow and its first time derivative. This parameterization is related to the LF model (Fant et al., 1985). At the end of this section the influence of different voice source parameters on these *flow waveshape parameters* is discussed.

The glottal flow waveshape can be subdivided into glottal open and closed period, and the open period itself can be subdivided into opening and closing period (Figure 4).

If the cartilaginous part of the glottis is completely closed, no glottal flow occurs in the closed period. The *leak flow* fl_{lk} reflects (i) the flow passing the cartilaginous part of the glottis together with (ii) the flow passing that part of the membranous glottis which never closes during the glottal (vibration) cycle. T_0 is the *duration of a complete glottal cycle* ($F0 = 1/T_0$). T_c represents the time instant of glottal closure and thus the *duration of the glottal open phase* equals T_c while the *duration of*

2 A strong increase in vocal fold tension is a further mechanism for controlling voicelessness (cf. Hanson and Stevens, 2002) beside increasing abducion. This mechanism will be considered in future modeling studies.

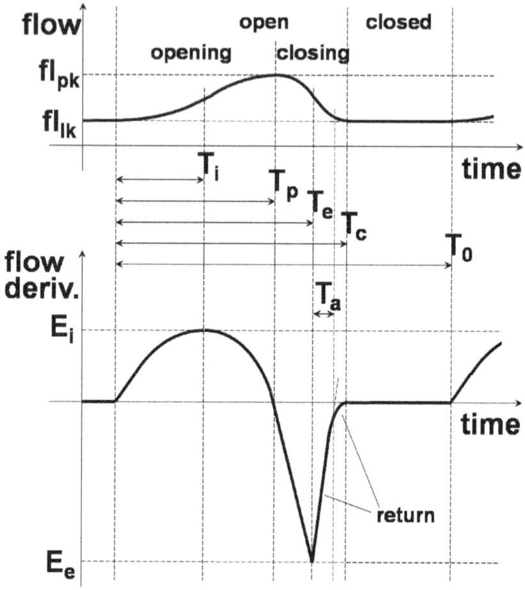

Figure 4. Typical waveshape of glottal flow and its first time derivative for one glottal vibration cycle in modal phonation. A description of the parameters is given in the text.

the closed phase can be calculated as $T_0 - T_c$. T_p represents the time instant of *peak flow* (or maximum flow) fl_{pk}. Thus the *duration of opening phase* equals T_p while the *duration of the closing phase* can be calculated as $T_c - T_p$. During the opening phase the time instant of maximum *increase* in glottal flow T_i can be identified and the maximum increase in flow is quantified as E_i. During the closing phase, in an analogous way the time instant of maximum *decrease* in glottal flow can be identified. This is the time point T_e, at which the voice source produces the *maximal vocal tract (acoustic) excitation*. The maximum (acoustic) excitation amplitude is given as E_e. The time interval between T_e and T_c is called the return phase and the *decay time* T_a as defined in Figure 4 is a measure for the *abruptness of glottal closure* (please note: $T_a < T_c - T_e$). If decay time T_a is zero, the glottis is closed in the most abrupt way by cutting down the flow to leak flow immediately at the time instant of maximum vocal tract excitation T_e. In this case the time derivative of glottal flow

abruptly decreases to zero at T_e. The more the decay time T_a increases, the less abrupt the glottal closure takes place. In this case the decay time T_a occurs between $T_c - T_e > T_a > 0$.
The *relative time parameters of the glottal flow waveshape* are always quantified relative to the length of the glottal cycle T_0 and thus relative to fundamental frequency. These parameters are RG, RE, OQ and RA in terms of the LF-model (Karlsson and Liljencrants, 1996): The *opening quotient* T_p/T_0 equals $1/2 * RG$, the *excitation time quotient* T_e/T_0 equals RE, the *open quotient* T_c/T_0 is also labeled OQ, and the *relative decay time* T_a/T_0 equals RA. In addition two glottal flow time parameters are quantified absolutely without being related to the voice fundamental. These are *opening frequency* FG, which equals $1/(2\pi T_p)$, and *decay frequency* FA, which equals $1/(2\pi T_a)$. The *open quotient* T_c/T_0 as well as the *flow pulse skewness* factor $(T_c/T_p) - 1$ (also labeled as *speed quotient* SP) give information about the waveshape of the vocal fold vibration. The relative location of the acoustic excitation time point with respect to the glottal opening period $(T_e/T_p) - 1$ is labeled as *excitation skewness* factor RK (Karlsson and Liljencrants, 1996), which is only slightly lower than flow pulse skewness since the time instant of maximal excitation T_e occurs at the end of the glottal pulse. *Peak flow* fl_{pk}, *leak flow* fl_{lk} (also called *dc-flow*), and the difference between peak flow and leak flow $fl_{pk} - fl_{lk}$ (also called *ac-flow*) are *aerodynamic parameters of the glottal flow wave shape* which can be used to adjust the vibrational amplitude of the vocal fold model and which can be used to adjust the aperture of the membranous and cartilaginous part of the vocal fold model x_m and x_c, if lung pressure is known. An interpretation of glottal flow parameters in terms of acoustics was put forward by Carlson et al. (1989). The main results are that fl_{pk} as well as E_i represent the amplitude or spectral energy of the voice fundamental. E_e (also sometimes labeled as EE) represents the spectral energy above FG. Both energy or amplitude levels should only be interpreted if they can be related to each other as $E(fl_{pk})/EE$ or E_i/E_e. The decay time T_a determines the spectral tilt of glottal flow (as well as of its derivative). Medium T_a around 0.15 ms (and higher values) leads to a medium spectral tilt of -12dB/octave for glottal flow. Medium T_a to minimum T_a around 0.0 ms leads to a less steep spectral tilt of about just 6dB/octave for glottal flow. Medium to maximum T_a of around 0.6 ms leads a steeper spectral tilt of about -18dB/octave for glottal flow.

From the simulation experiments done by Titze (1989a) it can be concluded even for our extended model that decay time T_a mainly increases with increasing vocal fold abduction x_m. Open quotient T_c/T_0 increases with vocal fold abduction but also with increasing converging glottal shape x_d and slightly with decreasing phase delay pha_v. But further simulation experiments will be done in this paper in order to highlight the relation between geometrical-articulatory and acoustic parameters of the voice source in more detail.

3 Laryngeal behavior of male and female breathy, modal, and pressed voice

Modal (or normal) phonation in the mid or mid-low region of the chest register means that the vocal folds (membranous part of the glottis) as well as the cartilaginous part of the glottis are nearly closed (x_m and x_c around 0). The peak-flow (fl_{pk}) and leak flow (fl_{lk}) are around 0.38 l/s (l=liter) and 0.12 l/s for males and around 0.22 l/s and 0.09 l/s for females (at lung pressure around 630 Pa for males and around 570 Pa for females, Holmberg et al. (1988)) indicating that a noticeable chink (i.e. a leak between the cartilaginous part of the glottis) exists for males as well as for female voices in the case of normal phonation. The flow waveform typically shows an open quotient T_c/T_0 of approximately 0.55 for male and around 0.75 for female voices (Holmberg et al., 1988; Klatt and Klatt, 1990; Karlsson and Liljencrants, 1996, and Table 2). The glottal pulse is slightly skewed with $(T_e/T_p) - 1$ as well as $(T_c/T_p) - 1$ of approximately 0.38 for male voices and 0.43 for female voices (Karlsson and Liljencrants, 1996). The spectrum of glottal flow has an average tilt of approximately 12 dB/octave (Klatt and Klatt 1990), and T_a is approximately 0.15 msec for male voices and around 0.2 msec for female voices (Karlsson and Liljencrants, 1996) and Table 2. Changing from modal to *pressed voice quality* means that the membranous and cartilaginous part and the glottis are now tightly closed and that a medial compression occurs at the vocal processes perpendicular to the length of the vocal folds (Klatt and Klatt, 1990). That leads to a narrowing of the glottal pulse and thus to a decrease in open quotient T_c/T_0 of about 0.41 for male voices, Karlsson and Liljencrants (1996) and Table 2). Glottal clo-

Table 2. Parameters of glottal flow shape and acoustic relevant parameters for male and female pressed (=P), modal (=M), and breathy (=B) voice after Karlsson and Liljencrants (1996). All parameters have been discussed in the text. SP is an abbreviation for skew of pulse (see text).

		MALE			FEMALE		
		P	M	B	P	M	B
F0 [Hz]	$(1/T_0)$	128	126	131	261	246	254
$1/2RG$ [%]	(T_p/T_0)	27.0	38.0	40.0	45.0	43.0	48.0
FG [Hz]	$(1/2T_p)$	229	167	164	289	284	266
RE [%]	(T_e/T_0)	39.2	52.0	60.5	67.6	65.8	71.0
OQ [%]	(T_c/T_0)	41.0	54.0	65.0	71.0	71.0	79.0
Ta [ms]		0.102	0.160	0.349	0.124	0.202	0.320
RA [%]	(T_a/T_0)	1.31	2.02	4.57	3.24	4.96	8.12
FA [Hz]	$(1/(2\pi T_a))$	1620	1001	461	1290	810	503
SP [%]	$((T_c/T_p)-1)$	39.5	37.7	51.1	50.0	51.8	48.5
RK [%]	$((T_e/T_p)-1)$	39.5	37.7	51.0	49.9	51.7	48.3

sure is more abrupt than in modal phonation. T_a is about 0.1 msec for male and female voices (Karlsson and Liljencrants, 1996) and Table 2 and consequently the spectral tilt is about -6 dB/octave for this change in voice quality. Leak flow (fl_{lk}) is about zero here due to a completely closed glottis during the closed period of the glottal cycle for male as well as for female voices. Changing from modal to *breathy voice quality* means that the arytenoids are well separated at their posterior end, but that the vocal processes (i.e. anterior end of the arytenoids) are sufficiently approximated so that the vocal folds are capable of vibrating. While vocal folds close simultaneously along their length during modal phonation, this is not the case in breathy phonation. Here the vocal folds first close at the anterior end and then the closure propagates towards the posterior end of the vocal folds (Figure 1a), leading to an overall flow waveshape with a rounded corner at the end of the return phase (Figure 4). That leads to an increase of T_a in comparison to modal voice (T_a is approximately 0.35 ms for male and female voices, Karlsson and Liljencrants (1996) and Table 2) and furthermore leads to an increase in the spectral tilt to approximately -18 dB/octave (Klatt and Klatt, 1990). It remains to mention that the anterior-posterior propagation of closure, which occurs for breathy voice, should not be confused with the inferior-superior propagation of glottal closure, which occurs for all voice qualities in chest register. Glottal closure always starts at the inferior part of the glottis and propagates towards the superior part and glottal opening starts from the inferior towards the superior part. This behavior also occurs for a strongly converging vocal fold configuration (large x_d). But in that case the closure does not occur along the whole inferior-superior dimension but only in the superior part of the glottal constriction. Notice that a converging pre-phonatory glottal shape is important in order to allow subglottal pressure to push apart the vocal folds from the inferior part of the glottal constriction and thus to start and to maintain vocal fold vibration.

4 Experiment: Synthesis of a male and female breathy, modal, and pressed voice quality

4.1 Motivation and hypothesis

The voice source model parameters of our voice source model and typical glottal flow parameters for pressed, modal, and breathy phonation for a male and female voice are introduced above (section 2 and section 3). It is the goal of this experiment to find adjustments of the model parameters of our voice source model such that it is capable of reproducing glottal volume flow waveshapes, which are comparable to those described by Karlsson and Liljencrants (1996) for male and female modal, breathy, and pressed voice quality (Table 2).

4.2 Method

A continuum of male and female phonatory or voice source states was generated by varying the degree of glottal abduction. A continuum was chosen since it is known that male and female voices differ in breathiness (Holmberg et al., 1988; Kröger, 1989; Klatt and Klatt, 1990). All states were generated by using a small male vocal tract positioned for a constant /a:/ (Birkholz and Kröger, 2006). F0 was adjusted to 126 Hz for the male and to 255 Hz for the female voice in order to produce voice source signals which are comparable with those reported by Karlsson and Liljencrants (1996) (see Table 2). In both sets of states (male and female), glottal abduction is varied from high negative values (representing a tightly closed glottis with medial compression on the vocal folds and thus with no occurrence of vocal fold vibration) to high positive values (voiceless sound condition and again no occurrence of vocal fold vibration). The cartilaginous part was assumed to abduct with a displacement value of x_c which is comparable to the displacement value of the upper (or superior) posterior part of the membranous part of vocal folds x_{mu} (see Figure 1). The variation of x_{mu}, which represents the continuum of varying degree of glottal abduction is listed in Table 3. Start-

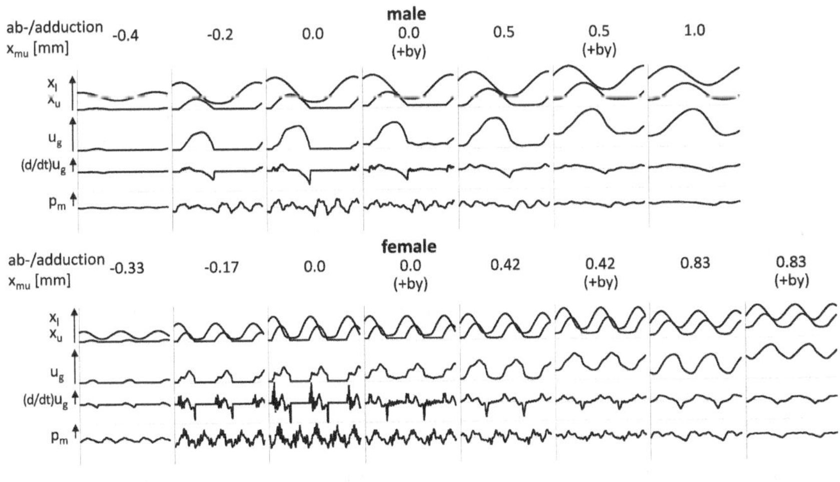

Figure 5. Waveshape of lower (inferior) and upper (superior) part of the vocal folds (distance x_l, x_u), of glottal flow u_g, of its first time derivative $(d/dt)u_g$, and of sound pressure radiated from the mouth p_m for approximately one glottal vibration cycle in the case of the male voice (upper row) and for approximately two glottal cycles in the case of the female voice (lower row) (time window is 10 ms in each case). Each row represents the continuum from pressed over normal towards breathy voice. The value given for each column is degree of ab-/adduction x_{mu} in mm (cf. Table 2).

ing with $x_{mu} = 0$, two cases can be separated: (i) increasing adduction towards $x_{mu} = -0.4$ mm for the male voice and towards $x_{mu} = -0.33$ mm for the female voice (see Table 3) and (ii) increasing abduction towards $x_{mu} = 1.0$ mm for the male and towards $x_{mu} = 0.83$ mm for the

Table 3. Parameters of glottal flow waveshape for (a) male and (b) female voices for different degrees of glottal ab-/adduction. The label (+by) indicates simulations including the cartilaginous part of the glottis (extended Titze 1984 model, see Birkholz 2005; the cartilaginous part is also labeled "aerodynamic bypass" or "+by"). All other cases represent simulations using the pure non-extended Titze (1984) model. No data indicate that no audible vocal tract excitation is generated in that case.

MALE								
ab-/adduct. ($x_m u$)	-0.4	-0.2	0.0	0.0 (+by)	0.5	0.5 (+by)	1.0	1.0 (+by)
$F0$ [Hz] $(1/T_0)$	127	126	126	125	124	126	125	-
$1/2RG$ [%] (T_p/T_0)	17.2	28.3	30.5	29.8	43.4	46.4	57.5	-
FG [Hz] $(1/2T_p)$	367	223	206	210	143	135	109	-
RE [%] (T_e/T_0)	24.7	44.0	48.6	48.6	63.1	62.7	80.2	-
OQ [%] (T_c/T_0)	31.3	46.3	50.3	50.0	71.1	72.5	93.6	-
T_a [ms]	0.476	0.181	0.068	0.087	0.399	0.658	1.036	-
RA [%] (T_a/T_0)	6.03	2.29	0.85	1.09	4.96	8.26	13.00	-
FA [Hz] $(1/(2\pi T_a))$	334	877	2340	1824	399	242	154	-
SP [%] $((T_c/T_p)-1)$	81.7	63.6	65.0	67.6	64.0	51.1	62.9	-
RK [%] $((T_e/T_p)-1)$	43.3	55.6	59.3	62.9	45.5	35.0	39.6	-
fl_{pk} [l/s]	0.018	0.180	0.272	0.292	0.378	0.460	0.453	-
fl_{lk} [l/s]	0.000	0.000	0.000	0.044	0.019	0.167	0.139	-
$fl_{pk} - fl_{lk}$ [l/s]	0.018	0.180	0.272	0.248	0.359	0.293	0.314	-
FEMALE								
ab-/adduct. ($x_m u$)	-0.33	-0.17	0.0	0.0 (+by)	0.42	0.42 (+by)	0.83	0.83 (+by)
$F0$ [Hz] $(1/T_0)$	256	255	255	253	256	255	256	257
$1/2RG$ [%] (T_p/T_0)	23.8	33.2	35.5	34.8	47.7	49.7	50.6	49.6
FG [Hz] $(1/2T_p)$	538	383	359	364	269	256	253	259
RE [%] (T_e/T_0)	33.1	45.7	49.7	49.4	66.3	67.6	70.1	67.1
OQ [%] (T_c/T_0)	37.2	47.4	51.4	51.7	73.3	76.3	81.4	80.2
T_a [ms]	0.159	0.065	0.045	0.057	0.162	0.312	0.420	0.476
RA [%] (T_a/T_0)	4.07	1.66	1.16	1.45	4.14	7.95	10.76	12.24
FA [Hz] $(1/(2\pi T_a))$	1003	2447	3509	2791	985	510	379	334
SP [%] $((T_c/T_p)-1)$	56.1	42.6	44.7	48.8	53.7	53.5	60.9	61.8
RK [%] $((T_e/T_p)-1)$	39.0	37.4	39.8	41.1	39.0	36.0	38.5	35.3
fl_{pk} [l/s]	0.039	0.125	0.160	0.198	0.241	0.312	0.297	0.408
fl_{lk} [l/s]	0.000	0.000	0.000	0.039	0.014	0.132	0.070	0.251
$fl_{pk} - fl_{lk}$ [l/s]	0.039	0.125	0.160	0.159	0.227	0.180	0.227	0.157

female voice (see Table 3 and Figure 5). For higher degrees of ab- or adduction no vocal fold oscillation occurs which is capable of exciting the vocal tract acoustically.
A slight inward rotation of the arytenoids was introduced by setting $x_c = x_{mu} + 0.25mm$ for the male and for the female voice if $x_{mu} \geq 0$. A further set of voice source states was generated in the case of abduction with $x_c = 0$ (case: no cartilaginous part i.e. non-extended Titze 1984 model; the other case is designated as "including aerodynamic bypass", abbreviated as "+by" in Table 3) for the male and female voice source. In all sets of states the glottis converges in the vertical direction from its inferior to its superior part (Figure 1b) and a convergence ratio $x_d/x_v = 3.0$ is assumed (this ratio varies between 1.0 and 5.0 according to Titze, 1989a). The glottal convergence parameter x_d was hold constant for all voice source states in all sets of states. Phase delay pha_v was set to 72° (see Titze, 1984) and kept constant within all sets. Lung pressure p_l was set to 630 Pa for males and to 570 Pa for females (see Holmberg et al., 1988, p. 525). Resulting waveshapes of the vocal folds, of glottal flow and its time derivative are shown in Figure 5. A quantitative estimation of time and flow parameters of our simulated voice qualities is given in Table 3.

4.3 Results

The parameter values listed in Table 3 indicate that vocal tract excitation occurs for glottal adduction until $x_{mu} = -0.4$ mm for male and until -0.33 mm for female voice and for glottal abduction until 1.0 mm for male voices (while in the case of an added cartilaginous part or "bypass" vocal tract excitation ends between 0.5 mm and 1 mm) and until 0.83 mm for the female voice. Concerning the glottal flow waveshape parameters and its acoustic consequences it can be stated: (i) Values of open quotient OQ increase from maximal adduction (negative values of x_{mu}) towards maximal abduction (positive values of x_{mu}) and OQ is always higher for the female than for the male voice for a given degree of ab-/adduction. These results are in accordance with natural data (e.g. Karlsson and Liljencrants, 1996). It can be concluded that an increase in glottal open period and consequently a decrease in glottal closed period indicates a change of voice quality towards breathy voice and vice versa a decrease towards pressed voice.

(ii) Values of opening quotient $1/2RG$ as well as values of reciprocal opening frequency $1/FG$ increase with increasing abduction and indicate an increasing opening period. But due to the parallel increase in open period this increase of opening quotient does not automatically result in an increase of pulse skewness. Values of pulse skewness SP of glottal flow resulting from our simulations are too high for the male voice and do not show the expected increase with decreasing adduction as it occurs in natural data (see Karlsson and Liljencrants, 1996). Only in the case of the female voice skewness values are comparable to natural data (ibid.). Thus in the natural case an increase in pulse skewness SP is expected for male and female voices if adduction increases (i.e. if the voice quality changes towards pressed voice). This tendency occurs in our simulations at least for the increase of glottal adduction between $x_{mu} = -0.2$ mm to $x_{mu} = -0.4$ mm in the case of the male voice and for the increase in glottal adduction between $x_{mu} = -0.17$ mm to $x_{mu} = -0.33$ mm in the case of the female voice.
(iii) As well as for open quotient also values of excitation time quotient RE increase from maximal adduction towards maximal abduction and these values are always higher for the female voice than those of the male voice for a given degree of ab-/adduction. These trends are in accordance with natural data (Karlsson and Liljencrants, 1996). Thus an increase of the excitation time quotient as well as an increase of the open quotient indicate a change of voice quality towards breathy voice and vice versa.
(iv) Excitation skewness RK values are too low in the case of the female voice in comparison to natural data (ibid.), but of the right order of magnitude in the case of the male voice. Excitation skewness naturally increases with increasing adduction. This is reflected in our simulations at least in the case of the change from breathy to normal voice (glottal adduction between $x_{mu} = 0.5$ mm and $x_{mu} = 0$ mm) for the male as well as for the female voice.
(v) Decay time parameters TA, RA, and reciprocal FA increase during glottal abduction while no clear tendencies can be found during glottal adduction for both the male and female voice. Values of decay TA are lower than 1.5 ms at $x_{mu} = 0$ for male as well as for female voices and above 1.5 ms in the case of abduction and this trend is in accordance with literature (Karlsson and Liljencrants, 1996; Klatt and Klatt, 1990). Only for strong adduction ($x_{mu} = -0.4$ mm for male and -0.33 mm

for female voice) a too high decay time value occurs in our simulations. The normally occurring decrease in *TA*, *RA* and reciprocal *FA* indicates a shallower spectral tilt of the voice source signal and thus an increase in amplitude of higher harmonics with increasing adduction.
(vi) Peak flow fl_{pk} and leak flow fl_{lk} are increasing during increasing abduction for all positive values of glottal ab-/adduction (i.e. in the case of normal to breathy voice). In the case of added bypass these values are even higher for a given degree of ab-/adduction. *AC*-flow $fl_{pk} - fl_{lk}$ is between approximately 250 l/s and 350 l/s for the male voice and between 150 l/s and 230 l/s for the female voice if glottal ab-/adduction values are positive (i.e. voice quality between normal and breathy voice). *AC* amplitude is still high in the case of high positive ab-/adduction values indicating that the audible signal fades away during abduction before the glottal vibration ends. These tendencies are in accordance with natural data (Holmberg et al., 1988). Thus vocal tract excitation fades away earlier than glottal vibration (amplitude) with increasing abduction from normal to breathy voice. For negative values of glottal ab-/adduction (i.e. in the case of the normal to pressed voice continuum) peak flow and *AC* flow decreases with increasing adduction and no leak flow occurs, which is in accordance with natural data as well (ibid.). Decreasing peak flow as well as AC flow in this case indicates the tendency of decreasing glottal opening with increasing adduction.

5 Discussion

The main result of this study is that our voice source model is flexible enough to cover the parameter ranges of voice source parameters that are defined by the LF model (Fant et al., 1985) for male and female pressed, modal, and breathy voice. Open quotient as well as opening and excitation time quotient as come out from our simulations of female and male voice cover the whole range of natural data (Karlsson and Liljencrants, 1996) and show the expected tendencies during abduction and adduction. Decay time, which reflects the spectral tilt of the source signal, also covers the range of natural data (ibid.) and shows the expected trends during abduction. Only in the case of strong adduction near the end of the breathy-normal-pressed continuum does decay time again increase, thus showing a too high value. Flow pulse skewness as well as excitation skewness values generated by the model do not show clearly the tendencies given in natural data. This may result from the strong ripple occurring with the glottal flow waveshape in the model as a consequence of glottal source vocal tract acoustic interaction (Bavegard and Fant, 1994) which makes it difficult to estimate the time instant of peak flow T_p in the case of the model flow waveshapes.

From the viewpoint of our model it would be possible in addition to vary not only glottal ab-/adduction as was done above but in addition to vary other parameters like phase delay pha_v (Titze, 1989a, p.197) as well as glottal convergence x_d (ibid.). But our experiments indicate that the parameter range for glottal flow parameters is sufficiently modeled by varying glottal ab-/adduction. Furthermore, varying bypass opening area A_c by varying width x_c and length L_c of the cartilaginous part of the glottis has an effect mainly on leak flow and decay time. But the value range for the acoustically important decay time is already sufficiently modeled by changing abduction of the membranous part of the voice source model. It can be concluded from these findings that the Titze (1984) model itself is capable of generating a wide spectrum of different glottal flow shapes and thus is capable of generating a wide value range of acoustically important flow parameters. But the addition of a bypass is important to adjust the overall flow and thus the aerodynamics of the mode which is, for example, important for the generation of frication noise in the vocal tract.

Our first perceptual impressions of the voice qualities generated by the model do not reflect the fact that the model is capable of generating the whole range of voice qualities along the breathy-normal(modal)-pressed continuum. Voice qualities always sound more or less modal. Only a slight effect towards breathy or pressed voice quality occurs even in the case of strong abduction and strong adduction. Two reasons may be responsible for this impression: (i) No glottal noise excitation source is implemented in our model. But the occurrence of glottal noise is important especially in the case of breathy voices (Klatt and Klatt, 1990). (ii) The waveshape of vocal fold vibration are always sinusoidal in the case of the Titze (1984) model since Titze (1984) by definition only allows sinusoidal waveshapes in his model. Only the amplitude and the phase lag can be varied for the vibration of the upper and lower part of the glottis. The sinusoidal character of waveshapes is reflected by unnaturally high decay time values in the case of high adduction. In order to overcome this disadvantage of the model (i) a glottal noise excitation source should be implemented in order to be able to generate convincing breathy voice quality and (ii) to increase the flexibility of possible waveshapes for vocal fold vibration by allowing to mix sinusoidal waveshapes with other types of waveshapes which in particular model very abrupt glottal closure in order to result in lower decay time values and thus higher excitation skewness. If it is the goal to avoid any presetting of a vocal fold waveshape, of its amplitude and of the phase lag between lower and upper part of the vocal folds, an alternative modeling approach would be to take the geometrical part of this model but to control the vocal fold vibration by a specific modeling of aerodynamic and mechanic forces, i.e. to combine the approach given in this paper with a self-oscillating vocal fold model (e.g. Liljencrants, 1996; Titze and Story, 2002; Drioli, 2005; Tao and Jiang, 2008).

6 Acknowledgements

This work was supported in part by the German Research Council Project Nr. Kr 1439/13-1 and project Nr. Kr 1439/15-1.

References

Badin, P., Bailly, G., Reveret, L., Baciu, M., Segebarth, C., and Savariaux, C. (2002). Three-dimensional linear articulatory modeling of tongue, lips and face, based on MRI and video images. *Journal of Phonetics*, 30(3):533–553.

Bavegard, B. and Fant, G. (1994). Notes on glottal source interaction ripple. *STL-QPSR, Royal Institute of Technology Stockholm*, (4):63–78.

Birkholz, P. (2005). *3D-Artikulatorische Sprachsynthese.* Logos-Verlag.

Birkholz, P., Jackèl, D., and Kroger, B. (2007). Simulation of losses due to turbulence in the time-varying vocal system. *IEEE Transactions on Audio, Speech, and Language Processing*, 15(4):1218–1226.

Birkholz, P., Jackèl, D., and Kroger, K. (2006). Construction and control of a three-dimensional vocal tract model. In *Proceedings of the IEEE International Conference on Acoustics, Speech and Signal Processing, Toulouse*, volume 1, pages 873–876.

Birkholz, P. and Kröger, B. (2006). Vocal tract model adaptation using magnetic resonance imaging. In *Proceedings of the 7th International Seminar on Speech Production, Belo Horizonte, Brazil*, pages 493–500.

Carlson, R., Fant, G., Gobl, C., Granström, B., Karlsson, I., and Lin, Q. (1989). Voice source rules for text-to-speech synthesis. In *Proceedings of the IEEE Conference on Signal Processing*, pages 223–226.

Chan, R. and Titze, I. (2006). Dependence of phonation threshold pressure on vocal tract acoustics and vocal fold tissue mechanics. *The Journal of the Acoustical Society of America*, 119:2351–2362.

Clark, R., Richmond, K., and King, S. (2007). Multisyn: Open-domain unit selection for the Festival speech synthesis system. *Speech Communication*, 49(4):317–330.

Drioli, C. (2005). A flow waveform-matched low-dimensional glottal model based on physical knowledge. *The Journal of the Acoustical Society of America*, 117:3184–3195.

Engwall, O. (2003). Combining MRI, EMA and EPG measurements in a three-dimensional tongue model. *Speech Communication*, 41(2):303–330.

Fant, G., Liljencrants, J., and Lin, Q. (1985). A four-parameter model of glottal flow. *STL-QPSR, KTH Stockholm, Sweden*, 4(1985):1–13.

Gobl, C. and Chasaide, A. (1988). The effects of adjacent voice/voiceless consonants on the vowel voice source: a cross language study. *STL-QPSR, KTH Stockholm, Sweden*, 2-3:23–59.

Gordon, M. and Ladefoged, P. (2001). Phonation types: a cross-linguistic overview. *Journal of Phonetics*, 29(4):383–406.

Hanson, H. and Chuang, E. (1999). Glottal characteristics of male speakers: Acoustic correlates and comparison with female data. *The Journal of the Acoustical Society of America*, 106:1064–1077.

Hanson, H. and Stevens, K. (2002). A quasiarticulatory approach to controlling acoustic source parameters in a Klatt-type formant synthesizer using HLsyn. *Journal of the Acoustical Society of America*, 112(3):1158–1182.

Hirano, M. (1983). The structure of the vocal folds. In Stevens, K. and Hirano, M., editors, *Vocal Fold Physiology.*, pages 33–43. University of Tokyo, Japan.

Hollien, H. (1960). Vocal pitch variation related to changes in vocal fold length. *Journal of Speech, Language and Hearing Research*, 3(2):150–156.

Hollien, H. and Moore, G. (1960). Measurements of the vocal folds during changes in pitch. *Journal of Speech, Language and Hearing Research*, 3(2):157.

Holmberg, E., Hillman, R., and Perkell, J. (1988). Glottal airflow and transglottal air pressure measurements for male and female speakers in soft, normal, and loud voice. *The Journal of the Acoustical Society of America*, 84:511–529.

Karlsson, I. (1992). *Analysis and synthesis of different voices with emphasis on female speech. (unpubl.)*. PhD thesis, KTH, Stockholm.

Karlsson, I. and Liljencrants, J. (1996). Diverse voice qualities: models and data. In *TMH-QPSR, KTH Stockholm, Sweden*, volume 2, pages 143–146.

Klatt, D. and Klatt, L. (1990). Analysis, synthesis, and perception of voice quality variations among female and male talkers. *Journal of the Acoustical Society of America*, 87(2):820–857.

Kröger, B. (1989). *Die Synthese der weiblichen Stimme unter besonderer Berücksichtigung der Phonation. (unpubl.)*. PhD thesis, Department of Phonetics, University of Cologne, Germany.

Kröger, B. (1993). A gestural production model and its application to reduction in German. *Phonetica*, 50(4):213–233.

Kröger, B. (1997). Zur artikulatorischen Realisierung von Phonationstypen mittels eines selbstschwingenden Glottismodells. *Sprache-Stimme-Gehör*, 21:102–105.

Kröger, B. (1998). *Ein Phonetisches Modell der Sprachproduktion*. Niemeyer, Tübingen.

Kröger, B. and Birkholz, P. (2007). A gesture-based concept for speech movement control in articulatory speech synthesis. In Esposito, A., Faundez-Zanuy, M., Keller, E., and Marinaro, M., editors, *Verbal and Nonverbal Communication Behaviours.*, pages 174–189. LNAI 4775, Springer, Berlin.

Kröger, B., Kannampuzha, J., and Neuschaefer-Rube, C. (2009). Towards a neurocomputational model of speech production and perception. *Speech Communication*, 51(9):793–809.

Liljencrants, J. (1996). Analysis by synthesis of glottal airflow in a physical model. . *TMH-QPSR, KTH Stockholm, Sweden*, 2:139–142.

Serrurier, A. and Badin, P. (2008). A three-dimensional articulatory model of the velum and nasopharyngeal wall based on MRI and CT data. *The Journal of the Acoustical Society of America*, 123:2335–2355.

Stevens, K. (1998). *Acoustic Phonetics*. MIT Press.

Story, B. and Titze, I. (1995). Voice simulation with a body cover model of the vocal folds. *Journal of the Acoustical Society of America*, 97:1249–1260.

Sundberg, J. (1987). *The Science of the Singing Voice*. Dekalb, Illinois.

Tao, C. and Jiang, J. (2008). A self-oscillating biophysical computer model of the elongated vocal fold. *Computers in Biology and Medicine*, 38(11-12):1211–1217.

Titze, I. (1984). Parameterization of the glottal area, glottal flow, and vocal fold contact area. *The Journal of the Acoustical Society of America*, 75:570–580.

Titze, I. (1988). The physics of small-amplitude oscillation of the vocal folds. *The Journal of the Acoustical Society of America*, 83(4):1536–1552.

Titze, I. (1989a). A four-parameter model of the glottis and vocal fold contact area. *Speech Communication*, 8(3):191–201.

Titze, I. (1989b). On the relation between subglottal pressure and fundamental frequency in phonation. *The Journal of the Acoustical Society of America*, 85(2):901–906.

Titze, I. (1989c). Physiological and acoustic differences between male and female voices. *Journal of the Acoustical Society of America*, 85:1699–1707.

Titze, I. and Story, B. (2002). Rules for controlling low-dimensional vocal fold models with muscle activation. *The Journal of the Acoustical Society of America*, 112:1064–1076.

The Role of Position in Testing the Acoustic-Equivalence Hypothesis of Velar Softening for Aspirated Stops

MARZENA ŻYGIS*
DANIEL RECASENS
AINA ESPINOSA

Abstract: Two hypotheses have been proposed in order to account for velar softening, i.e., a process in which /k/ changes to a sibilant affricate. Whereas one hypothesis states that for the process to apply the velar stop has to be realized as an (alveolo)palatal stop (articulation-based hypothesis), the other claims that velar softening is triggered by acoustic similarity between the input and output segments (acoustic-equivalence hypothesis). The present paper investigates the acoustic-equivalence hypothesis by comparing several acoustic properties of /k/ in various vowel contexts with those of /t͡s, t͡ʃ, t͡ɕ/ in languages differing in stop burst aspiration, i.e., German, Polish and Catalan where voiceless stops are strongly aspirated, slightly aspirated and unaspirated, respectively, and by testing perceptually whether the stop can be identified as a palatal affricate or a palatal fricative. Results suggest that the acoustic-equivalence hypothesis could account for velar softening in aspirated velar stops but not in unaspirated velar stops. This hypothesis was tested perceptually by presenting aspirated /k/ stimuli recorded by a German speaker to German and Catalan subjects for identification. Results show that the acoustic-equivalence explanation may hold provided that the stop occurs in intervocalic position where burst frication may be especially prominent and the burst spike may be severely reduced. Affricate identification percentages were found to be higher for Catalan speakers, who produce unaspirated stops, than for German speakers with aspirated stops in their consonant system.

* Dear Bernd, when I first met you several years ago, I did not have the faintest idea that you would guide me on my path to Habilitation via M.A. thesis and Ph.D. thesis. You gave me the freedom to research and warned me against the potential cul-de-sacs. Thank you very much, Bernd, for putting so much time and effort into constructive criticism of my work. Due to your trust in my grasp of phonetics, I could develop my interest in the phonetics-phonology interface. Last but not least, we all learn from you how to combine science and humanity in the most optimal way. Marzena

1 Introduction

Velar Softening, i.e., the change of a velar stop into /t͡ʃ/ or /t͡s/ is a widely attested process which takes place in various vowel contexts. For instance, according to the First Slavic Velar Palatalization /k/ changed to /t͡ʃ/ before /j/ and front vowels. The subsequent Second Slavic Velar Palatalization converted /k/ to /t͡s/ before short /e/ and short /i/ (cf. Carlton, 1991). In addition to the Slavic languages, Velar Softening is also frequently found in Romance (e.g., Italian [ˈtʃɛnto] "one hundred" from Latin /ˈkɛnto/), Bantu and other language families (English *chin*, *child* from Old English *cinn*, *cild*; Lass 1994, p.55).
Two explanatory hypotheses have been proposed in order to account for this sound change. First, velar softening has been explained on an articulatory basis by claiming that it is triggered by particular anterior, (alveolo)palatal realizations of the velar stop in several contextual and positional conditions, but also before low vowels and word finally presumably through articulatory strengthening. In fact, the articulation-based hypothesis has been the only available hypothesis for several decades (Rousselot, 1924-1935; Scripture, 1902; Grammont, 1971; Anttila, 1972; Hock, 1986). The other, more recent hypothesis (Chang et al., 2001; Guion, 1996, 1998; Ohala, 1992) claims that velar softening is associated with acoustic equivalence between the spectral cues for a front velar stop, i.e., a velar stop before a front vowel or glide, and the resulting affricate. In these circumstances, the stop burst shows a long /ʃ/-like frication noise with a 2500-3500 Hz spectral peak, and both front /k/ and /t͡ʃ/ are accompanied by rising F2 vowel transitions.
Production and perception data for Majorcan Catalan (Recasens and Espinosa, 2009) suggest that velar softening for unaspirated velar stops has an articulatory origin. CV stimuli containing the burst of the unaspirated (alveolo)palatal stop allophone [c] of underlying /k/ and some portion of the following vowel could be identified as /t͡ʃ/ by Catalan informants, more often when the stop preceded a low back vowel than when it preceded a high front vowel which is in line with the prominence of the burst energy and the vowel transitions in the former vowel context, and fairly often when the stop occurred word-finally. This result may account for the replacement of /k/ by /t͡ʃ/ via [c] in the same or similar conditions in Romance dialects and other language families

where [c] is present either as a phoneme or as an allophone of /k/. Guion (1998) has shown that analogous stimuli with English aspirated front velar stops may be heard as /t͡ʃ/ when mixed with high intensity white noise. A reason why /k/ before /j, i, e/ was better perceived as an affricate when aspirated than when unaspirated may be because aspirated stops exhibit longer and perhaps more intense bursts than unaspirated stops. A possible objection to Guion's study is that the presence of too low a signal-to-noise ratio in her stimuli could have caused a significant increase in the number of /t͡ʃ/ identification responses, i.e., the acoustic-equivalence hypothesis worked out to some extent only if the white noise was superimposed on the stimuli. The two above studies (Guion, 1998; Recasens and Espinosa, 2009) agree that an increase in the acoustic prominence of the stop burst contributes to higher affricate identification percentages.
Within this framework, this paper seeks to shed light onto the acoustic factors causing front /k/ to be confused with /t͡ʃ/ and other affricates in languages and dialects lacking [c] and exhibiting different degrees of stop burst aspiration:

1. German, where velar stops are strongly aspirated,
2. Polish, where they are slightly aspirated, and
3. Eastern Catalan, where they are unaspirated.

The main hypothesis is that strongly aspirated front /k/ should be more prone to be heard as /t͡ʃ/ than moderately aspirated front /k/ while unaspirated front /k/ should yield essentially no /t͡ʃ/ responses. The paper will be divided into two sections, one devoted to the production data analysis, and the other to the perceptual testing of the initial hypotheses.

2 Production

2.1 Methodology

Data include the stop sequences /kj, ki, kɛ, ka, kɔ, ku/ as a possible palatalization output, and the affricate sequences /t͡sa, t͡ʃa/ and, in ad-

dition, /t͡ɕa/ for Polish. Affricates may exhibit language-dependent differences in place of articulation: /t͡s/ is dental in Polish, dentoalveolar in German and centroalveolar or even postalveolar in Catalan; /t͡ʃ/ is postalveolar in German, postalveolar or alveolopalatal in Catalan, and apico-postalveolar in Polish where it is also called 'retroflex'; Polish /t͡ɕ/ is alveolopalatal. It is predicted that the burst acoustic prominence will be higher for /kj, ki, kɛ/ than for the other sequences and that, judging from the frequency of application of velar softening in synchronic and diachronic processes, it will be higher for /kj/ than for /ki/ and for /ki/ than for /kɛ/ (cf. typological study on /t/ palatalization in Hall et al. (2006)).
Two German, two Polish and two Catalan speakers read a set of controlled, short sentences with bisyllabic words including the sequences of interest in stressed word-initial position. The words were inserted in the following sentences:

1. German: *Ich habe __ gesagt* (7 syllables) 'I have __ said.'
2. Polish: *Powiedziala __ do niego* (9 syllables) 'She said __ to him.'
3. Catalan: *Ell deia __ fort* (6 syllables) 'He was saying __ loud.'

Recordings were performed at 44 kHz and downsampled to 20 kHz for analysis. Several acoustic cues for stops were submitted to analysis:
(i) Frequency of the front-cavity dependent burst spectral peak on autocorrelation LPC spectra using a 25 ms full-Hamming window and 14 coefficients. The window was centered at the onset of the frication noise immediately after the burst spike for stops, and at the midpoint of the frication period for affricates. Fronting closure location for the stop should cause the frequency of the burst spectral peak to increase, thus approaching the noise spectral peak of /t͡ʃ/.
(ii) VOT duration, which is equivalent to the burst duration since it was obtained by adding up the durations of the burst spike, the following burst frication period, and the burst aspiration period wherever available.
(iii) Burst absolute intensity, as well as burst relative intensity with respect to the intensity level of the adjacent vowel. Intensity values were taken at the same frame selected for measuring the spectral peak frequency. The intensity of the burst frication noise increases with airflow

volume velocity, and is also determined by front-cavity size at stop release (and thus especially high before low and back vowels in the case of velar stops; Dorman et al. 1977).
(iv) Endpoints and ranges of the F2 and F3 vowel transitions. Formant frequency measurements were taken in 10 ms steps placing a cursor in the middle of the formants, and on LPC spectra if spectrographic readings were judged not to be reliable enough. The frequency ranges of the vowel formant transitions were computed by subtracting the frequency values at the endpoint of the formant transitions from those obtained at the midpoint of the vowel.
As for affricates, measures included the spectral peak frequency and intensity of the frication noise, duration of the burst spike + frication noise, as well as the endpoints and ranges of the vowel transitions.
ANOVAs with repeated measures were performed on the measures (i) through (iv) for the /kV/ sequences across languages with 'vocalic segment' as the only factor (there were not enough data to run two-factor repeated measures ANOVAs with 'language' as a factor). The factor levels were 'j, i, ɛ, a, ɔ, u'. Each of the six speakers under analysis contributed one averaged score per condition. Huynh-Feldt corrected degrees of freedom were applied and Bonferroni post-hoc tests were run on the significant effects. The degree of significance was set at $p<0.05$.

2.2 Results

2.2.1 VOT

As shown in Figure 1, VOT values for /k/ vary in the progression German (80-115 ms) > Polish (35-65 ms) > Catalan (25-65 ms), and are significantly higher for /j, i/ than for non-high vowels ($F(3.7, 18.6) = 15.76$, $p<0.001$). The duration of the frication period for all affricates is about 85-125 ms, except for Polish apico-postalveolar /t͡ʃ/ which shows a short 50 ms frication period.

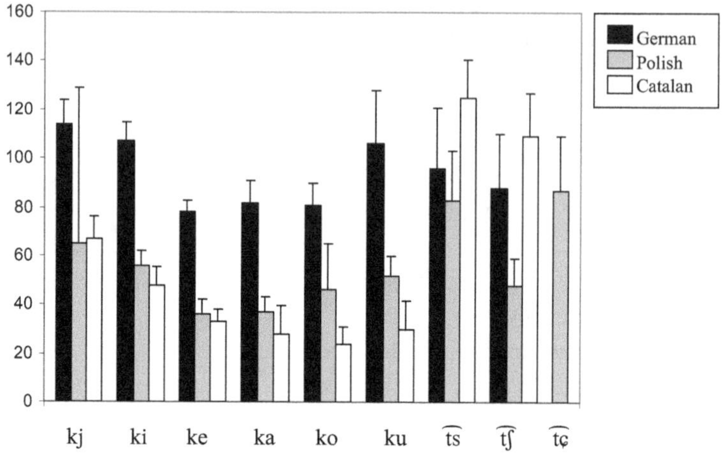

Figure 1. VOT in ms. Error bars in this and all other figures correspond to +/-1 standard deviation.

2.2.2 Burst spectral peak

The burst spectral peak frequency is comparable across languages and yielded highly significant contextual effects ($F(5, 25) = 188.00$, $p<0.001$). According to results from post-hoc tests, frequency values decrease significantly with vocalic context in the following progression (see Figure 2): /j, i/ (2850-3250 Hz) > /ɛ/ (1900-2350 Hz) > /a/ (1600-1800 Hz) > /ɔ/ (1050-1150 Hz) > /u/ (750-900 Hz). The burst peak frequency for /t͡ʃ/ (2600-3500 Hz) resembles that of /kj, ki/, while that for /t͡s/ is located at a much higher frequency in German and Polish (6500-7500 Hz) than in Catalan where the alveolar fricative is known to be apical and exhibit a palatalized quality (3750 Hz). The Polish affricate /t͡ɕ/ has an intermediate burst spectral frequency between that for the two other affricates (4000 Hz).

2.2.3 Transition endpoint

Analogously to the burst spectral peak, the F2 transition endpoint frequencies are comparable across languages and yielded significant contextual effects ($F(2, 10.2) = 86.56$, $p<0.001$). According to results from post-hoc tests and as shown in Figure 3, contextual differences vary for

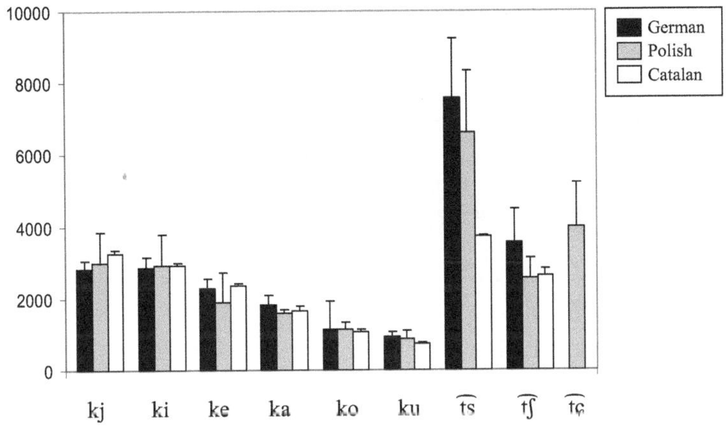

Figure 2. Burst spectral peak (in Hz).

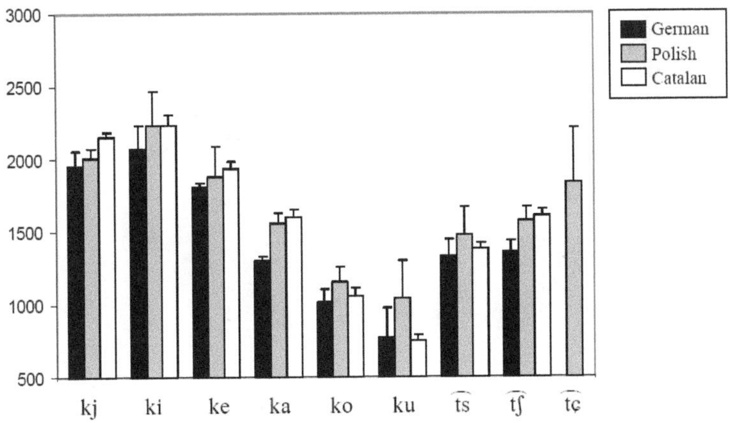

Figure 3. F2 transition endpoint (in Hz).

/j, i/ (1950-2250 Hz) > /ɛ/ (1800-1950 Hz) > /a/ (1300-1600 Hz) > /ɔ, u/ (750-1150 Hz). Regarding the F3 vowel transition endpoints, significant results were obtained for /j/ and, less so, /i/ (2700-3200 Hz) vs. the other vowels (2100-2500 Hz) ($F(3.7, 18.6) = 18.79$, $p<0.001$). The F2 transition endpoints for the affricates resemble those of /k/ in the context of /a/ (/t͡ʃ/ = 1350-1600 Hz; /t͡s/ = 1350-1500 Hz) while those for /t͡ɕ/ are higher (1850 Hz), see Figure 3. As for the F3 transition endpoints, the affricate shows intermediate values between /kj, ki/ and /ka/ (/t͡ʃ, t͡s/ = 2250-2600 Hz, /t͡ɕ/ = 2550 Hz).

2.2.4 Transition range

F2 transition ranges turned out to be significantly larger in the context of /j/ (+450 to 675 Hz) than in those of all other vocalic segments (-100 to +300 Hz) ($F(2.9, 14.6) = 23.69$, $p<0.001$), cf. Figure 4.

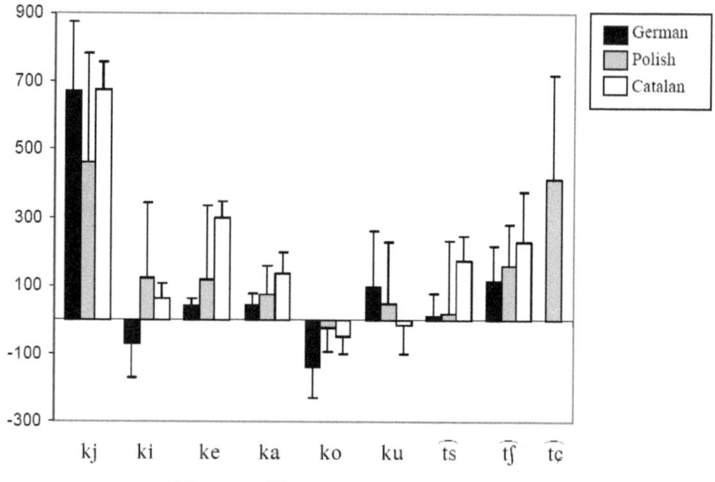

Figure 4. F2 transition range (in Hz).

They were also large and positive for /ɛ, a/, at least in Catalan. F3 transition ranges were also significantly larger in the context of /j/ ($F(3.2, 16) = 9.49$, $p<0.001$). Positive F2 transition ranges for the affricates /t͡ʃ/ and /t͡s/ next to /a/ were less prominent than those for /kj/ and more similar to those for /ki, kɛ/, i.e., 0 to +225 Hz.

2.2.5 Intensity

Context-dependent effects on absolute and relative stop burst intensity turned out to be non-significant, though mean values happened to be somewhat higher for non-high (55-65 dB) compared to high (52-60 dB) vocalic segments, cf. Figure 5.

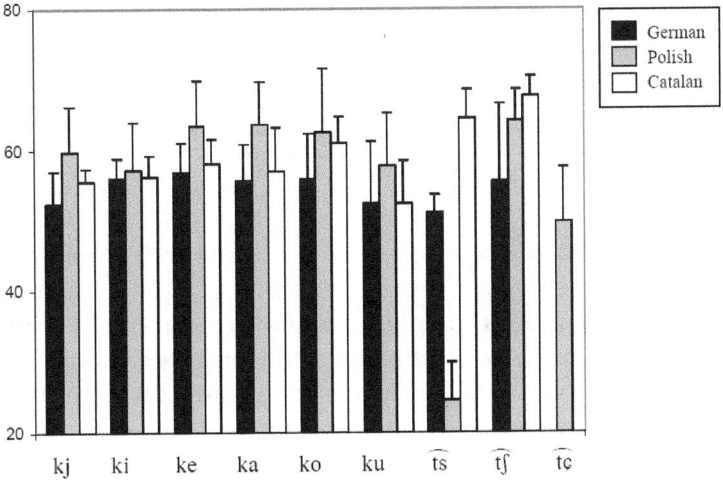

Figure 5. Absolute intensity (in dB).

These contextual differences are in agreement with differences in front cavity size for the two vowel types (see section 2.1). Values for /t͡ʃ/ and, less so, for /t͡s/ are similar to the highest intensity values for /k/ in the context of /a/ in German and Polish, i.e., about 50-65 dB (absolute) and 0.70-0.80 (relative). In Catalan, the two affricates are more intense than the stop, i.e., about 65 dB (absolute) and 0.95 (relative).

2.3 Summary

Based on VOT values for /k/ and affricates reported in the Results section, it appears that, at least at the production level, German aspirated front velar stops are more prone to be integrated as affricates than their slightly aspirated or unaspirated cognates in Polish and Catalan. Burst intensity level is also similar for both stops and affricates in German. Moreover, the burst frequency peak and the transition endpoints and ranges vary with the following vocalic segment in the progression front > low > back rounded, thus indicating that the replacement of /k/ by /t͡ʃ/ ought to take place mostly before /j/, and more so before /i/ than before /ɛ/. Long-range vowel transitions for the sequence /kj/ are associated with the gliding nature of /j/.

In principle, these findings would be in support of the acoustic-equivalence hypothesis stating that aspirated velar stops ought to change to affricates due to acoustic similarity between the input and output segments. The acoustic-equivalence hypothesis could also provide an explanation as to why aspirated velar stops are prone to undergo softening more easily when followed by /j, i, ɛ/ than by /a/ or schwa, or word finally.

The articulation-based hypothesis, on the other hand, would apply to unaspirated velar stops which are expected to yield /t͡ʃ/ via the (alveolo)palatal stop [c]. Accordingly, a preliminary perceptual evaluation of the sequences submitted to analysis in the present paper reveals that Eastern Catalan unaspirated front velar stops cannot be identified with affricates, which leads us to hypothesize that velar softening can only be triggered by (alveolo)palatal stop realizations in this case. This would also answer the question why softening of unaspirated velar stops may take place not only before front vowels and glides but also before low and central vowels as well as word finally where a prominent burst and/or large formant frequency ranges appear to favour the process application.

3 Perception

In looking for an acoustic explanation of velar softening for aspirated stops, we listened to short CV excerpts of tokens of word-initial /ki, kj/ produced by several German speakers (those whose data were analyzed in the preceding section) to see whether they could be categorized as CV sequences with an alveolopalatal affricate. The word-initial position was chosen because it is supposed to be the most prominent position of all and therefore should contribute to affricate perception. The excerpts in question paralleled those used in previous work on velar softening (Guion, 1998; Recasens and Espinosa, 2009) in that they were composed of the stop closure, the stop burst and 100 ms of the following vowel. The two first authors (MZ: Polish speaker and DR: Catalan speaker) failed to categorize the aspirated front velar stop as an affricate. This result suggests that, unless white noise is superimposed on the excerpts of interest (see Introduction), front /k/ cannot be integrated as /t͡ʃ/ even if aspirated. In principle, this would also imply that, analogously to unaspirated stops, velar softening for aspirated velar stops is triggered by articulatory variations.

We then hypothesized that the failure of the acoustic-equivalence account to work out might have been due to the fact that the most natural position for velar softening in the case of aspirated stops may not be the word-initial position after a pause but the intervocalic position, whether occurring word medially (VCV) or across a word boundary (V#CV).

The rationale for this expectation is to be found in the intensity level of the stop burst. Perception data for unaspirated (alveolo)palatal stop allophones of /k/ reveal indeed that the stop is likely to be heard as /t͡ʃ/ with an increase in the burst noise intensity level, and that this perceptual effect occurs more clearly in VCV than #CV sequences (Recasens and Espinosa, 2009). These perception data are consistent with acoustic data showing a higher noise intensity and more prominent transition ranges in intervocalic than word-initial position (a similar spectral peak frequency occurs in both positions). Data from the literature also show that stop burst and vowel intensity in CV sequences with aspirated stops increases with stress (Cho and McQueen, 2005), and that velar softening for unaspirated stops is more likely to operate in stressed vs. unstressed position (Friulian [ˈt͡ʃazɛ] CASA 'house', [kaˈmiŋ] CAMINU 'path'; Jaberg and Jud, 1928-1935).

In addition to burst intensity, it may be that velar softening is more prone to apply intervocalically than postpausally because consonants may undergo articulatory reduction in the former position but not in the latter. Lenition causes aspirated voiceless stops to change into voiceless fricatives since vowel opening triggers undershoot in closure formation and burst implementation. For a stop to become a fricative, the burst spike must cease to be perceived. The closure period may shorten. In these circumstances, it seems that front velars could yield a palatal-like frica-

tive. One could also hypothesize that, if closure for reduced aspirated stops is still relatively long (though shorter than for non-reduced stop productions), a palatal affricate may be heard.
Support from sound change processes may be adduced in support of our hypothesis, i.e., fricativization through weakening affects voiceless stops mostly if they are velar or uvular (/k/ > [x, h], /q/ > [χ]; Lavoie (2001, p.32). In specific areas of the Gorgia Toscana, the change /k/ > [x, h] occurs more often than /p/ > [ɸ] and /t/ > [θ] in intervocalic position both within the word and across words (Villafaña Dalcher, 2006).
In summary, acoustic equivalence could account for aspirated velar stop softening in intervocalic position through a decrease in intensity of the stop burst spike and perhaps through an increase in intensity of the burst frication noise. In order to explain why velar softening affects word-initial /k/ so often, it may be hypothesized that, since the change started out intervocalically in V#CV sequences, it occurred word initially as well.
Two tests were performed in order to verify the validity of this formulation of the acoustic-equivalence hypothesis. First, a comparison was carried out between the intensity level and duration of the burst frication portion for aspirated front /k/ in word-initial and intervocalic position. Second, a perception test was run in order to check whether decreasing the burst spike intensity value in successive steps would contribute to identifying aspirated front /k/ as /t͡ʃ/ or /ʃ/.

3.1 Position effect

In order to test the acoustic-equivalence hypothesis we prepared a new set of data containing words with /ki/ and /kj/ in word-initial and intervocalic position. Word-initial /k/ was placed in utterance-initial position since we wanted to highlight the prominence of the velar stop burst. We chose German as the testing language due to its strong stop aspiration. Two native speakers of German (JD, male and MB, female) read the following set of randomized sentences 10 times each. In addition, the same set of data was read by both speakers putting emphasis on the words given in boldface so as to ensure that /k/ would be louder and exhibit a longer aspiration period.

word-initial position

/ki/	**[ki]ra** ist heute gekommen. 'Kira has come today.'	(8 syllables)
/kj/	**[kj]ara** ist heute gekommen. 'Chiara has come today.'	(8 syllables)

intervocalic position

/i#ki/	Er hat d[i **ki]ra** vorgestellt. 'He has introduced Kira.'	(8 syllables)
/i#kj/	Er hat d[i **kj]ara** vorgestellt. 'He has introduced Kjara.'	(8 syllables)

Recordings were performed at 44 kHz and downsampled to 20 kHz for analysis. The acoustic analysis was conducted using PRAAT. The following two parameters were submitted to analysis using the same procedure as described in section 2:

1. Duration of VOT, i.e., the acoustic period including burst spike, frication and aspiration.

2. Absolute intensity of the burst frication period, and corresponding relative intensity with respect to the intensity level of the adjacent vowel.

Figure 6 presents VOT values for /ki/ and /kj/ in word-initial and intervocalic position obtained from speakers JD and MB. The longest VOT corresponds to intervocalic /ki/ (speaker JD: 90 ms; speaker MB: 95 ms). Moreover, VOT is longer in intervocalic vs word-initial position for /ki/ (both speakers) and for /kj/ (speaker JD). A two-tailed t-test revealed that the VOT value for /k/ is longer intervocalically than word initially in the context of /i/ but not of /j/ for both speakers (speaker JD: $p<0.01$; speaker MB: $p<0.05$).
As far as absolute intensity is concerned, a position-dependent significant difference was found to hold only for /kj/ (46.09 dB) vs. /ikj/ (53.26 dB) as produced by speaker JD ($p<0.001$). Similarly, relative intensity, i.e., the ratio of the absolute intensity of the burst frication noise with respect to the intensity of the following vowel, turned out to be significant for the same sequences /kj/ vs. /ikj/ produced by JD ($p<0.001$),

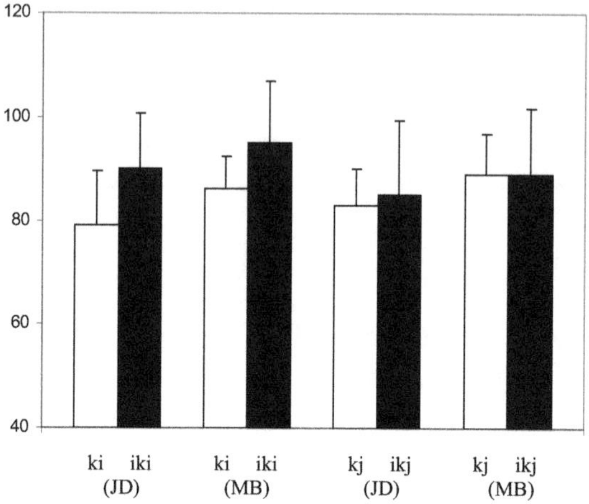

Figure 6. VOT (in ms).

cf. absolute and relative intensity values in Figure 7 and 8, respectively. Our calculations also reveal that emphasis does not affect burst duration or intensity, i.e., no significant differences in VOT or intensity were found to occur between the emphatic and non-emphatic productions. We assume that speakers may use other cues such as vowel duration or pitch for emphasizing syllables. In summary, our acoustic investigation shows differences in VOT between word-initial and intervocalic position, i.e., longer VOT values for /iki/ than for /ki/ for both speakers. Intensity appears to set /kj/ and /ikj/ in contrast for one speaker (JD) with again the intervocalic position being marked by stronger intensity levels than the word-initial one.

3.2 Perception test

The speaker MB's token of /iki/ exhibiting the highest burst amplitude was chosen for preparing the acoustic stimuli of a perception test. In the token in question, the aspirated velar stop had a 77.5 ms closure, a 16 ms burst spike and an 88 ms frication period. The stop burst spike was attenuated from 53 dB down to 35 dB in 3 dB steps, thus yielding seven stimuli overall. The frication period of the stop burst was left

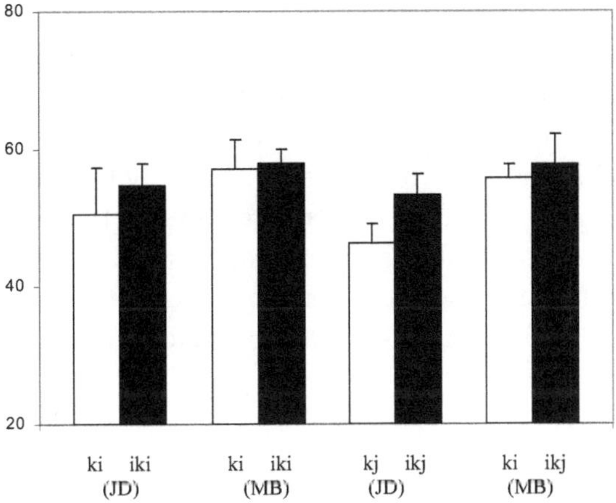

Figure 7. Absolute intensity (in dB).

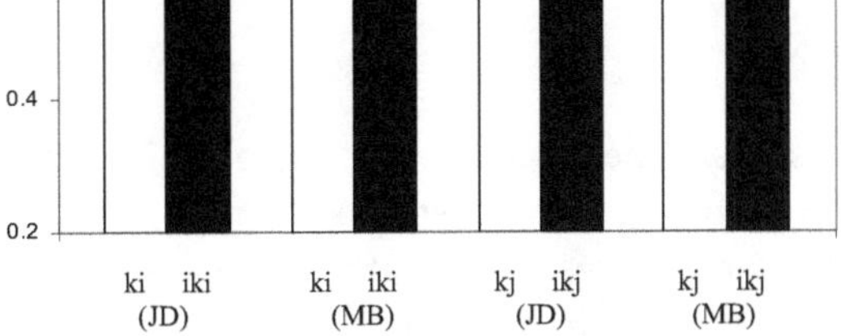

Figure 8. Relative intensity (in dB).

unmodified. A perception test was prepared which included seven tokens of each stimulus and thus, 49 tokens. The stimuli were randomized and presented for identification. 15 German and 9 Catalan subjects were asked to identify the stop excerpts as /k/ or as /t͡ʃ/ or /ʃ/ by writing the appropriate orthographic symbols on an answer sheet. Data for /t͡ʃ/ and /ʃ/ were computed jointly since very few fricative responses were elicited (we will thus refer to /t͡ʃ/ responses only from here onwards). Mean affricate identification percentages are plotted in Figure 9 as a function of stimulus number and language as well as across languages. Stimulus amplitude values proceed from 35 dB (stimulus 1) to 53 dB (stimulus 7) in 3 dB steps. According to the identification curves in the

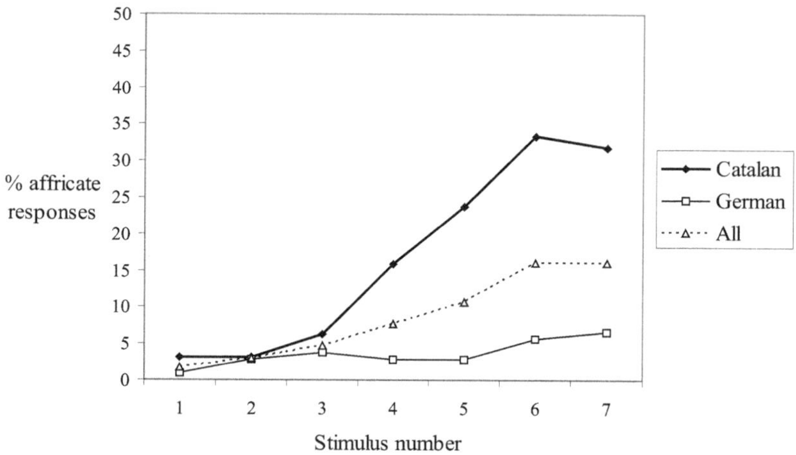

Figure 9. Affricate identification percentages.

figure, Catalan subjects heard aspirated /k/ as /t͡ʃ/ about 30-35% in the case of stimuli exhibiting low burst spike intensity values. As for German, maximum percentages are about 5%. It thus appears that Catalan subjects were more ready to categorize /k/ as an affricate. Moreover, data for the individual subjects indicate that only a few of them could hear aspirated /k/ as /t͡ʃ/, i.e., three out of nine Catalans and only one out of fifteen Germans.

4 Discussion and conclusions

Analysis and perception data reported in this paper reveal that velar softening may be attributed to different factors, i.e., articulatory variation for unaspirated stops and acoustic equivalence for aspirated stops. It should be noticed that the articulatory account could also be at the origin of velar softening for aspirated stops.

A relevant finding of this paper is that the acoustic-equivalence explanation appears to hold only if the stop occurs in intervocalic position where burst frication may be particularly prominent and the burst spike may be severely reduced. A reduction in burst spike intensity level combined with the presence of a short closure may trigger the perception of /k/ as /t͡ʃ/.

Affricate identification percentages were found to be higher for Catalan speakers who produce unaspirated stops than for German speakers with aspirated stops in their consonant system. It thus appears that the former subjects paid more attention to the frication component than the latter precisely since their stop productions show no aspiration. The perception behaviour of the Catalan subjects was by no means unanimous, however, since two thirds of them could not categorize the perception stimuli as affricates.

5 Acknowledgements

We would like to thank Jörg Dreyer for technical support, Matthias Ziervogel for his help in conducting the perceptual experiment with German subjects, Phil Hoole and an anonymous reviewer for comments. This research has been supported by projects GWZ-4/11-1-P2 of the German Research Foundation, 01UG0711 of the Federal Ministry of Education and Research of Germany, HUM2006-03742 and FFI2009-09339 of the Ministry of Education/Innovation and Science of Spain and FEDER, and 2005SGR864 and 2009SGR003 of the Catalan Government.

References

Anttila, R. (1972). *An Introduction to Historical and Comparative Linguistics.* MacMillan, New York.

Carlton, T. (1991). *Introduction to the Phonological History of the Slavic Languages.* Slavica Pub, Columbus, Ohio.

Chang, S., Plauché, M., and Ohala, J. (2001). Markedness and Consonant Confusion Asymmetries. In Hume, E. and Johnson, K., editors, *The Role of Speech Perception in Phonology.*, pages 79–101. Academic Press, New York.

Cho, T. and McQueen, J. (2005). Prosodic influences on consonant production in Dutch: Effects of prosodic boundaries, phrasal accent and lexical stress. *Journal of Phonetics*, 33(2):121–157.

Dorman, M., Studdert-Kennedy, M., and Raphael, L. (1977). Stop-consonant recognition: Release bursts and formant transitions as functionally equivalent, context-dependent cues. *Perception and Psychophysics*, 22(2):109–122.

Grammont, M. (1971). *Traité de phonétique.* Delagrave, Paris.

Guion, S. (1996). *Velar Palatalization: Coarticulation, Perception and Sound Change.* PhD thesis, University of Texas at Austin.

Guion, S. (1998). The role of perception in the sound change of velar palatalization. *Phonetica*, 55(1-2):18–52.

Hall, T., Hamann, S., and Zygis, M. (2006). The phonetic motivation for phonological stop assibilation. *Journal of the International Phonetic Association*, 36(01):59–81.

Hock, H. H. (1986). *Principles of Historical Linguistics.* Mouton de Gruyter, Berlin.

Jaberg, K. and Jud, J. (1928–1935). *Sprach- und Sachatlas Italiens und der Südschweiz (AIS), 6 Vol.* Universität Zurich, Zofingen.

Lass, R. (1994). *Old English: A Historical Linguistic Companion.* Cambridge University Press, Cambridge.

Lavoie, L. (2001). *Consonantal Strength. Phonological Patterns and Phonetic Manifestations.* Garland, New York.

Ohala, J. (1992). What's Cognitive, What's not, in Sound Change. In Kellermann, G. and Morrisey, D., editors, *Diachrony within Synchrony: Language History and Cognition.*, pages 309–335. Peter Lang Verlag, Frankfurt.

Recasens, D. and Espinosa, A. (2009). Acoustics and perception of velar softening for unaspirated stops. *Journal of Phonetics*, 37(2):189–211.

Rousselot, J.-P. (1924-1925). *Principes de phonétique expérimentale.* Welter, Leipzig.

Scripture, E. (1902). *The Elements of Experimental Phonetics.* Charles Scribner's Sons, New York.

Villafaña Dalcher, C. (2006). *Consonant Weakening in Florentine Italian. An Acoustic Study of Gradient and Variable Sound Change.* PhD thesis, Georgetown University, Washington.

Schwa Deletion under Varying Prosodic Conditions: Results of a Pilot Study *

CHRISTIAN GENG
CHRISTINE MOOSHAMMER
HOSUNG NAM
PHILIP HOOLE

Abstract: Pretonic schwa elision, as in e.g. *support* → *sport*, has been conceptualized as a change in intergestural timing by Articulatory Phonology (Browman and Goldstein, 1994). This study aims at a preliminary evaluation of predictions made by the current version of the theory (Saltzman et al., sub) by comparing C_1 C_2 coordination in bisyllabic /C_1əC_2VC/words with monosyllabic /C_1C_2VC/ words: In order to address this question we recorded the tongue and lip movements of two speakers of British English by means of EMA. Both speakers showed the predicted longer lag between the first two consonants in words like *police* than in *please*. The first consonant was not integrated into the syllable in the pretonic schwa condition. Furthermore, we tested whether the schwa in pretonic position has a specified vowel target. The movement of the tongue dorsum suggests that the trajectory is determined by the context, at least for one speaker. This would support a targetless schwa interpretation.

1 Introduction

There has been a growing body of evidence in support of the idea that temporal patterns in speech production are an essential characteristic of phonological organization. Especially, the fact that many phonological processes, such as final devoicing, vowel neutralization and assimilation, seem to be gradual rather than categorical lends evidence to this

* Thanks to our mentor whose nickname has stimulated the design of the current experiment.

view. In this study, we want to explore further whether temporal variation alone can explain the phenomenon of pretonic schwa deletion. Impressionistically, the schwa in the first syllable of words such *police* appears to be deleted in fast speech (see Hooper, 1978; Kaisse, 1985, for a recent overview see Davidson, 2006). For many words, such as *tomorrow* $\rightarrow$ *tmorrow*, pretonic schwa deletion yields consonant sequences that are phonotactically illegal. However, a number of studies found that schwa deletion is not a categorical process with the schwa being either deleted or not, but rather varies continuously in duration and quality (e.g. Jannedy, 1994, after Beckman 1996).

Apart from the question of the categoricalness versus the graduality of the process that relates representations with and without a schwa or not, the exact nature of representation has also been debated. A related topic is whether the perceived schwa has its own specification for place of articulation, or whether it results from the timing relations between the surrounding consonants and their articulatory specifications. In the latter case the quality of this so-called transitional schwa would be determined completely from the surrounding consonants, and - even more interestingly from a phonological point of view - would not be there underlyingly.This approach, which runs counter to most phonological theories, accounts for the fact that schwa deletion is not a categorical process but a continuous process varying on a hyperarticulation continuum. One pole of this continuum is occupied by a hyperarticulated version with a substantial delay between the two consonants, which is transformed into the other pole by a gradual increase in overlap in such a way that the first syllable eventually loses its syllabicity.

The variation between these two extreme forms of timing was modeled within the framework of Articulatory Phonology (Browman and Goldstein, 1990a) as a continuous stepwise change in the timing between the two consonants. Timing relations between gestures account for e.g. reduction phenomena (Browman and Goldstein, 1990b), syllable related allophony in laterals and nasals (for an overview see Krakow, 1999) and the properties of consonant sequences in different syllable positions (Browman and Goldstein, 2000). In earlier versions of Articulatory Phonology, intergestural timing was specified manually or based on rule; however, more recently, a planning model of intergestural timing has been developed (Browman and Goldstein, 2000; Nam and Saltzman,

2003; Goldstein et al., 2010). In this model, gestures are associated with planning oscillators and pairwise coupled to one another, which constructs a coupling network of gestures, called coupling graph. Steady-state relative phases from coupled oscillators are used to trigger relative timing among gestures, which is timing between gestural onsets. The coupling graphs (see Saltzman et al., 2008) can be organized on several prosodic levels which control the organization of linguistic material in a more principled way than was possible in the older versions of AP. In the model, vowel and consonant gestures are coupled with one another in two basic modes (in-phase and anti-phase), which are spontaneously available without difficulty (Haken et al., 1985) or the necessity for repetitive practice. In CV sequences, the consonant and vowel gestures are coupled to each other synchronously or in phase, and in VC sequences the consonant and vowel gestures are sequentially coupled with a 180°phase-lag or so-called anti-phase coupling. Note that this kind of coupling is also assumed for consonant sequences. Based on studies by Byrd (1996), Honorof and Browman (1995), Browman and Goldstein (2000), and others, the timing of consonant sequences differs with respect to their position in the syllable. The organization of /C_1C_2VC/ material is assembled by the onset consonants' competing tendencies to be coupled in-phase to the vowel and anti-phase to each other. The resulting compromise shifts the phasing of the onset material from 180° in consonant sequences in codas or across boundaries to 120° (C-centre timing, see Figure 1 on the following page). This is in contrast to /C_1C_2VC/ with a reduced initial syllable. The timing between C_1 and C_2 is sequential, which corresponds to 180°. In absolute terms it depends on the reduction introduced by the prosodic modulation gesture (Saltzman et al., 2008). Additionally the fact that schwas are colored by the consonantal context to a much greater degree than unreduced vowels can be modeled via shortening due to a prosodic modulation gesture. For the bisyllabic case, as in *police*, two different variants have been suggested, with and without an underlying schwa. The first one to discuss here assumes that the schwa in the pretonic syllable is specified for TBCL (tongue body constriction location) and TBCD (tongue body constriction degree), i.e. the schwa has a target of its own (for the assumption of a lexical schwa see e.g. Smorodinsky, 2002). As shown in Figure 2 the timing relation between the initial stop and the lateral in e.g. *police*

<please>

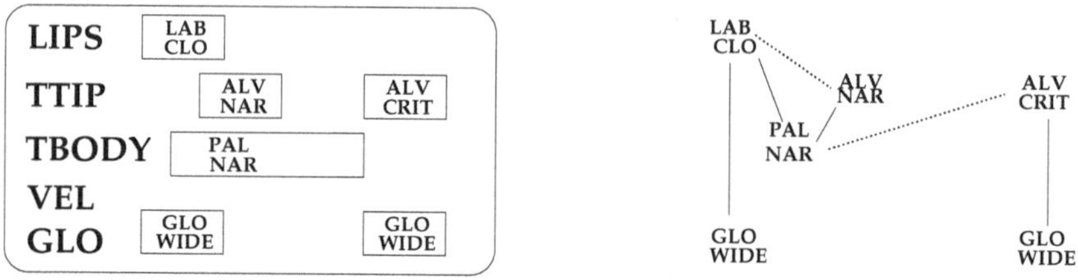

Figure 1. Illustration of C-centre timing in complex onsets (120°). In-phase couplings are shown as solid lines, anti-phase couplings as dotted line. Explanations of Gestural CL/CD specifications: LAB CLO - Labial Closure, PAL NAR - Palatal Narrowing, ALV NAR/CRIT - Alveolar narrowing / critical constriction, GLO WIDE - Glottis wide.

is anti-phase even though they are not directly linked. The initial /p/ is initiated synchronously with the schwa, i.e. a 0° in-phase coupling; the schwa is timed sequentially with the following syllable, i.e. a 180° anti-phase coupling. Evidence for an underlying schwa with its own TBCL and TBCD gestures comes from Browman and Goldstein (1994); they found tongue dorsum troughs during the schwa in sequences such as /pipəpip/. One possible explanation for the apparent contradiction between Browman and Goldstein's papers (1990a and 1994) could come from the effects of the segmental context (stop-liquid versus stop-stop environments) as hypothesized in Browman and Goldstein (1990a).[1]

The second modeling variant with a transitional schwa has been suggested by several researchers, e.g. Browman and Goldstein (1990a) and Davidson (2006) for American English. According to their hypothesis, *bray* and *beret* are distinguished only by their gestural organization but not by the number of gestures. As shown in Figure 3, even without an explicit vowel gesture in the first syllable the timing between /p/ and /l/ is sequential, which is the default cross-syllable phasing. Again, shortening of the pretonic syllable can be modeled by applying a prosodic modification gesture to the reduced syllable.

Therefore, the two representations in Figures 2 and 3 do not differ in their phasing specification but in the fact that for the first representation

1 The paper that appeared later (Browman and Goldstein, 1994) actually seems to predate the older work in Browman and Goldstein (1990a).

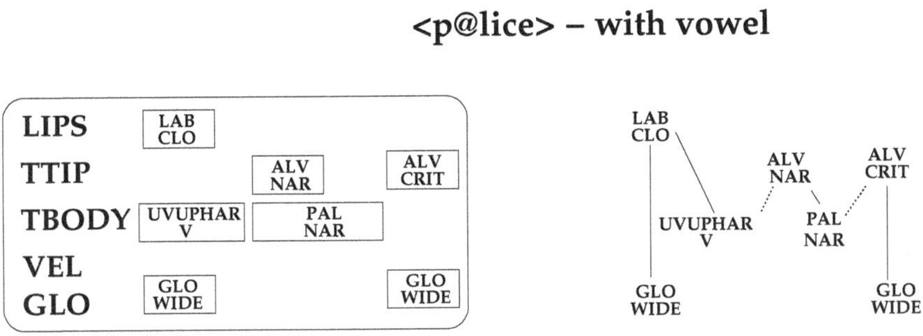

Figure 2. Gestural Score and coupling graph in /C$_1$əC$_2$VC/. The example word is represented with a reduced initial syllable. This representation contains a lexical schwa but is otherwise identical to Figure 3.

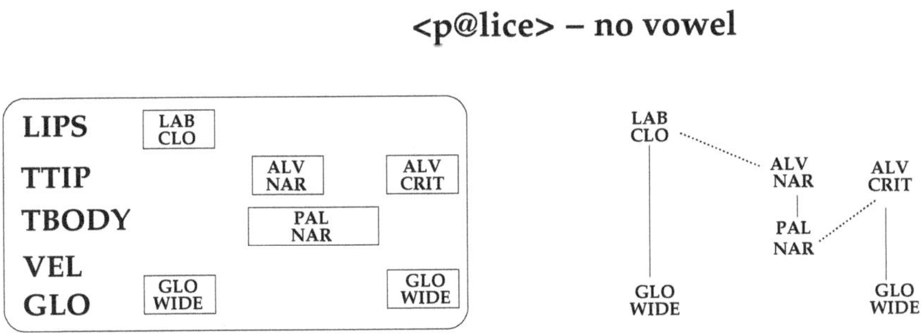

Figure 3. Gestural Score and coupling graph in /C$_1$əC$_2$VC/ with a reduced initial syllable. This variant has no lexical schwa.

we expect the tongue dorsum to move towards a vocalic target whereas for the targetless schwa the tongue dorsum trajectory during the labial and tongue tip gestures is completely determined by the consonantal context. Browman and Goldstein (1990a) informally stated that they did not observe differences in tongue dorsum movement shape during the interval between the bilabial and /r/ in words like *beret* and *bray*.

In the current study we aim at testing empirically whether speech production data give evidence for a targetless schwa or for a specified vowel gesture in pretonic position. Furthermore, the timing between the first consonants in word pairs such as *police* and *please* is investigated. Our assumption is that we will find a longer lag between the first two consonants in the pretonic reduced syllable than between the consonants when forming an onset cluster. We expect this difference in timing to be stable across prosodic conditions or speech rates. Temporal variation in this study was introduced by varying sentence accent which should shorten the delay for reduced syllables to a greater degree than for onset clusters which are known to be very stable (see Byrd, 1996).

2 Method

2.1 Experimental Procedure

We recorded articulatory motions of two native speakers of British English by means of articulography (EMA AG500, Carstens Medizinelektronik, c.f. Hoole et al. 2003, Hoole and Zierdt 2010 for more detailed descriptions of the method). The system is designed to track articulatory motion over time by attaching sensors to various locations in the vocal tract. Three sensors were attached midsagittally to the tongue: the front-most sensor (TT) was positioned roughly 1cm behind the actual tongue tip, the rearmost sensor (TB) as far back as possible without creating discomfort for the participant, and the third sensor (TM) such that its distance from TM and TB was roughly equal. Articulatory data were acquired at a sample rate of 200 Hz. Position estimation was done with the help of the TAPAD toolbox (see Hoole and Zierdt, 2010). The data were low-pass filtered before and after position estimation with FIR filters (Kaiser window): First, the raw amplitude data were filtered, and, after position estimation, the same filter was applied again to the position estimations before head correction. For the reference sensors (right and left ear, bridge of nose and maxilla), the filter cutoff was set to 5 Hz, for the TT to 40 Hz and to 20 Hz for all the other sensors (including the two rear tongue sensors, lips and jaw). After position estimation, the contributions of head movement were removed from the measured data on a frame-by-frame basis. Horizontal, vertical and tangential velocities were calculated using a filter that was obtained by convolving a differentiation kernel with filter coefficients of a lowpass filter with 20 Hz passband and 30 Hz stopband edges respectively (again using a Kaiser window). Audio data were simultaneously captured at a sampling rate of 32 kHz with an AKG CK98 shotgun microphone.

2.2 Stimuli

Currently we have collected data from two native speakers of British English, with no known history of speech, hearing or language problems reported. Three series consisting of real words were recorded (S1: *balloon bloom boon loon*, S2: *police please peace lease*, S3: *collapse claps caps laps)*. The main focus is on /$C_1əC_2$/ in comparison to the complex onset condition /C_1C_2/, whereas the monosyllabic words with singleton C_1 and C_2 onsets are used as control conditions in the C-centre analyses.

Table 1. Experimental items. Material belonging to the onset is shown in bold face; the consonant used as anchor point is printed in *italics*.

Test Items		
Series	Condition	Item
b/l	Elision	**balloo***n*
	Cluster	**bloo***m*
	C_1	**boo***n*
	C_2	**loo***n*
p/l	Elision	**poli**ce
	Cluster	**plea**se
	C_1	**pea**ce
	C_2	**lea**se
p/l	Elision	**colla***p*se
	Cluster	**cla***p*s
	C_1	**ca***p*s
	C_2	**la***p*s

In contrast to most previous studies weakening of the neutral vowel was elicited by prosodic manipulation: The target words were manipulated by an accent variation, i.e. they were recorded in an accented condition and a postnuclearly deaccented condition. For elicitation, two sentences were simultaneously displayed on the prompting screen, with the first one read in silence, and the second - the target sentence - read aloud. For example, the screen presentation for an accented item was "What did you say? I said a POLICE again" and for an deaccented item "Was it the larger police? No, it was the NICER police again." In total, six items were recorded in each condition. In the unaccented condition, the order of the words "nicer" and "larger" that conditioned contrastive stress was balanced: We recorded three repetitions in which "larger" occurred in the (unread) prompting question and "nicer" occurred in the test sequence itself, and also three repetitions per condition in which this order was interchanged. Table 1 gives an overview over the stimulus material acquired.

2.3 Data labelling

For each constriction movement, a number of elementary temporal landmarks were extracted. They are displayed in Roman numerals in Figure 4.

CLOSING MOV ON (I)	The onset of the movement towards the constriction was extracted using a 20% velocity criterion.
CONSTR ON (II)	The beginning of the constriction phase.
MAX CONSTR (III)	The point of maximum constriction was operationalized as the maximum in the vertical displacement signals.
CONSTR OFF (IV)	The end of the constriction phase.

These elementary landmarks were used to define additional point landmarks:

C1MID/C2MID:	were defined as the middle of the closure phase of each consonant, i.e. the timepoint temporally equidistant to the CONSTR ON and CONSTR OFF landmarks of the respective constriction gestures. This particular point was chosen because it turned out that it is more stable than the point of maximum constriction.
C-centre	was in turn defined as the duration between the midpoint of the interval [C1MID to C2MID] and the anchor point.
ANCHOR:	is an alias for the constriction onset of the coda consonant (CONSTR ON).

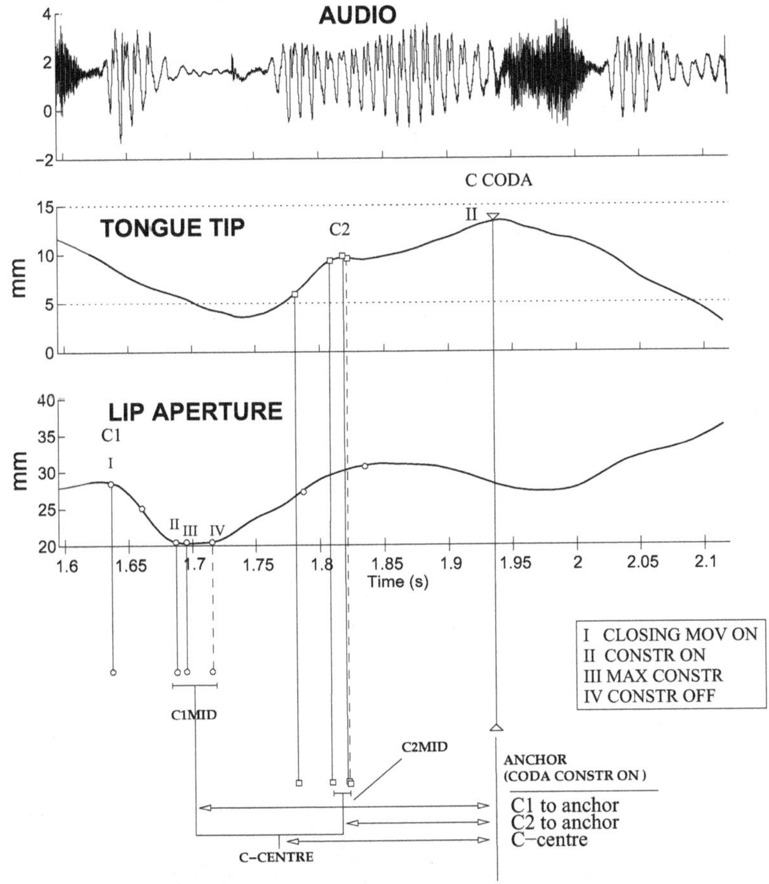

Figure 4. Illustration of the data labelling procedure an instance of the testword *police*. For each constriction, landmarks I to IV were extracted semi-automatically: CLOSING MOV ON (I), CONSTR ON (II), MAX CONSTR (III), CONSTR OFF (IV). The definitions of composite intervals are illustrated below the figures, (i) the duration between the first onset consonant and the consonantal anchor ("C_1 to anchor"), (ii) the duration between the second onset consonant and the anchor ("C_2 to anchor") and (iii) the C-centre.

These will serve to compute the dependent variables analysed in this contribution, i.e. measures of constriction overlap of initial consonants and durations of various consonantal landmarks to ANCHOR. The measure of constriction overlap analysed here is adopted from Hoole et al. (2010) and consists in the time between the end of the first consonant's constriction (C1 CONSTR OFF) and the time of onset of the nucleus of the second consonant (C2 CONSTR ON). This time interval can be analysed in absolute terms (in ms). Alternatively, it can be normalized by the time between the beginning of the first consonant's nucleus constriction (C1 CONSTR ON) and the end of the second gesture's constriction (C2 CONSTR OFF), and in the letter case yields a percentage. The interpretation of this measure is that increasingly positive values correspond to increasing overlap of C_1 and C_2, and negative values convey the information that the constriction phases show a lag between the consonants. As was addressed in the introduction, onset consonants show neither in-phase nor anti-phase timing with the following vowel but a compromise timing, called C-centre. This measure was calculated as the duration between the midpoint of the interval [C1MID to C2MID] and the anchorpoint later in the syllable. The C-centre of onset clusters should be aligned with the centre of a singleton in a CVC word.

3 Results

The following description will describe the differences between consonant sequences with and without an intervening schwa. This section is organized such that first temporal and then spatial patterns will be assessed (sections 3.1 and 3.2). Section 3.1 is further subdivided: In the first part we will describe the temporal organization of the onset consonant sequence material itself (section 3.1.1). After that the C-Centre will be introduced and discussed (section 3.1.2). Section 3.2 will investigate whether and how tongue dorsum movements differ for the two conditions.

3.1 Transconsonantal timing

3.1.1 Constriction overlap

Results for the patterns of absolute constriction overlap are shown in Figure 5. As described in section 2.3, constriction overlap is defined as the time between the end of the constriction nucleus of the first consonant (C1 CONSTR OFF in Figure 4) and the time of onset of the constriction of the second consonant (C2 CONSTR ON in Figure 4). As can be seen in Figure 5, the two consonants are always separated, i.e. the two constriction target regions do not overlap. In the case of the intervening schwa the absolute lag is consistently longer than for the cluster. The accent condition did not consistently affect the patterns of constriction overlap. This finding is somewhat unexpected, since the manipulation of accent was introduced in order to trigger schwa deletion – instead of the speech rate manipulation used in previous research on this topic. This issue will be considered again in the discussion section.
Interestingly, the variability of intergestural timing, measured as standard deviations in Figure 5, shows no tendency to be lower for the onset cluster than for the pretonic schwa syllable. This is the opposite to what could have been expected from previous studies on the behaviour of onset clusters (e.g. Byrd, 1996).
In summary, it was found that onset clusters were produced with a consistently shorter lag than consonant sequences with an intervening schwa which gives evidence against a complete homophony of the onsets of e.g. *police* and *please*.

3.1.2 Durations to anchorpoint: C-centre

This section describes observed patterns of timing of the consonantal onset material with respect to a consonantal anchor point in the rhyme. The consonantal anchor point was the rhyme consonant's constriction onset, i.e. the CONSTR ON marker. The CONSTR ON marker was chosen empirically by a stability analysis comparing candidate anchor points involving the centre of the rhyme consonant and the timepoint of the rhyme consonant's maximal constriction in addition to the CONSTR ON marker. The method of stability analysis was adopted from Shaw et al. (2009) and consisted in the the comparison of the coefficients of

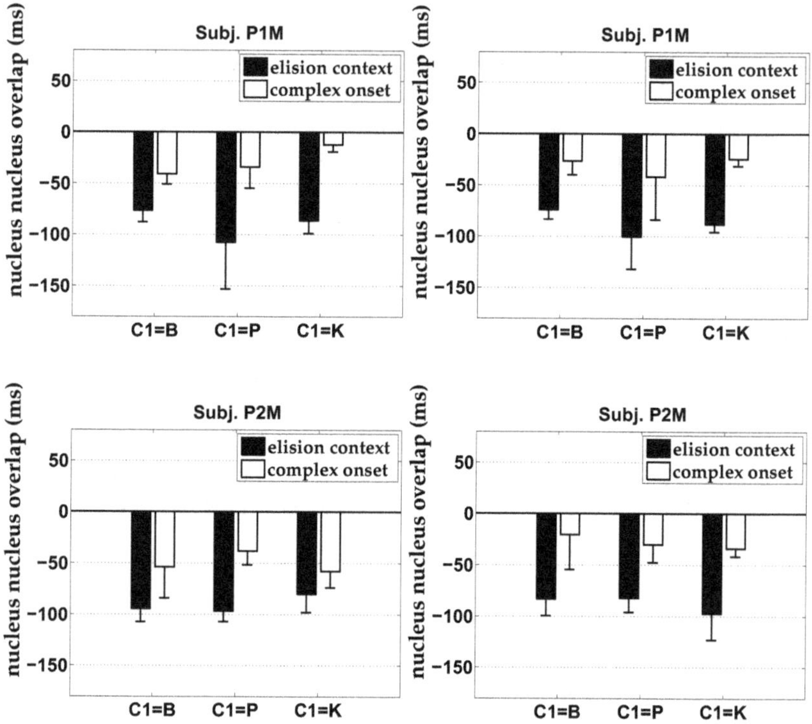

Figure 5. Plots of absolute constriction overlap of complex onset consonants and elision context respectively, both for the accented condition (left panels) and unaccented conditions (right panels). Speaker P1M is shown in the top row, speaker P2M in the bottom row. More negative values correspond to longer lags between C_1 and C_2.

variation (also called relative standard deviations) across the candidate anchors. It turned out that the constriction onset was marginally more stable according to this analysis. For singletons, the graphs in Figures 6 and 7 display the durations between the onset consonant's temporal midpoint to the anchor point in the rhyme as defined above. For elision contexts and consonant clusters, both C_1 and C_2 consonants' temporal midpoints, and in addition the C-centre are displayed relative to the consonantal anchor.

Figures 6 and 7 show the syllable timing relationships for participant P1M and P2M. Missing data for speaker P1M (C2 singletons for the test word *lease*, series *police*) are caused by annotation problems. Movement amplitudes of the tongue tip in the syllable onset consistently were too small to extract all necessary landmarks.

For the data to conform to the C-Centre hypothesis, the C-Centres in cluster contexts (shown as plus-signs in Figures 6 and 7, second row) should align with the singletons (shown as circles in Figures 6 and 7). This effect should be independent of the particular identity of the onset consonant in the singleton, i.e. C_1 and C_2 should show the same duration to the anchorpoint which means that the circles for the singletons in Figures 6 and 7 should align. For the elision context, the triangles (i.e. the second consonant) should be aligned with the singletons because C_2 /l/ is also the onset of the second syllable, at least in the absence of effects of polysyllabic shortening: An interpretation in terms of polysyllabic shortening would make two interrelated predictions. First, the interval between the second onset consonant and the anchorpoint should be shorter for the elision context than both for the cluster conditions and the singleton conditions. Second, it would make the same predictions for the C-Centre for the singletons considered alone, i.e. there should be no difference between C_1 and C_2 to anchorpoint durations. Deaccentuation should have a uniform effect of shortening the interval between the C-Centres and the anchorpoint because of the potential of the stressed vowel to undergo shortening.

The observations can be summarized as follows: The probably most eye-catching pattern in our data is that the C-Centre of the cluster and the singletons (the circles) do not align well in most cases. This is mainly because the C_2-singleton to anchorpoint durations are shorter in most cases (except in P2M's unaccented *police* series). The alignment with the

C_1-singleton is slightly better in accordance with the C-Centre hypothesis, but still the data do not warrant a fully consistent interpretation. The C-centres of the pretonic syllables precede the ones of clusters for most series. This effect is significant if a t-test is calculated over all data ($t = 3.05$, $df = 111.6$, $p < 0.01$). It fails to reach the level of significance though if speaker P1M's data are considered alone. This is due to the accented items of the *police* series and the unaccented items of the *collapse* series for which the C-centres of the elisions are actually closer to the anchorpoint than for the clusters. The patterns for speaker P2M are more consistent, but interestingly the pattern is attenuated for the same experimental condition (the accented *police* series, see Figure 7, top left panel). Still, in general this result can be interpreted as the expected failure to integrate the initial stop into the syllable in words with pretonic syllables.
A second observation is that there is a tendency for the durations between the second consonant – i.e. the /l/– and the anchorpoint - to be shorter for the lexically bisyllabic elision contexts (as denoted by the triangles) than for the other conditions. Again there are exceptions consisting in the C_2 accented clusters of *balloon* (P1M) and the *collapse* series (P2M). The shorter C_2 to anchorpoint interval for the pretonic condition in comparison to the clusters could reflect shortening of the following stressed vowel due to polysyllabic (foot) shortening (Turk and Shattuck-Hufnagel, 2000; Saltzman et al., 2008).

3.2 Spatial organization

In addition to the analysis of temporal patterns we also attempted to analyze the spatial patterns in order to compare the lingual behaviour during pretonic syllables and clusters in the different accent conditions. In order to arrive at a qualitative description, we calculated ensemble averages for the tongue mid sensors. For deaccentuated cases, we averaged over the different carrier phrases (see the stimulus description in section 2.2). The choice of the tongue mid sensor was motivated by the fact that it should, in contrast to tongue back and tongue front sensors, minimize segment-specific coarticulatory contributions from neighboring sounds. It is therefore considered the most appropriate sensor for the analysis

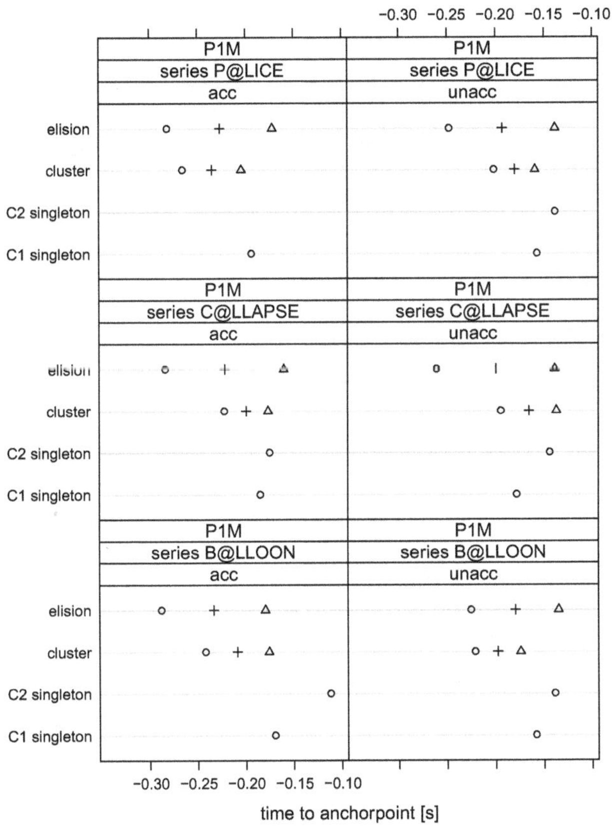

Figure 6. Lags to the rhyme anchor point for onset consonant material, speaker P1M. For singletons the analysis comprises the onset consonant's temporal midpoint. For elision context and consonant clusters, both onset consonants' temporal midpoints are displayed, and also the additional C-centre. The circles represent the initial consonants' midpoints. For elision and cluster contexts, plus-signs and triangles represent the C-center and the rightmost consonant's midpoint. Note there are missing data in the *police* series (see text for explanation).

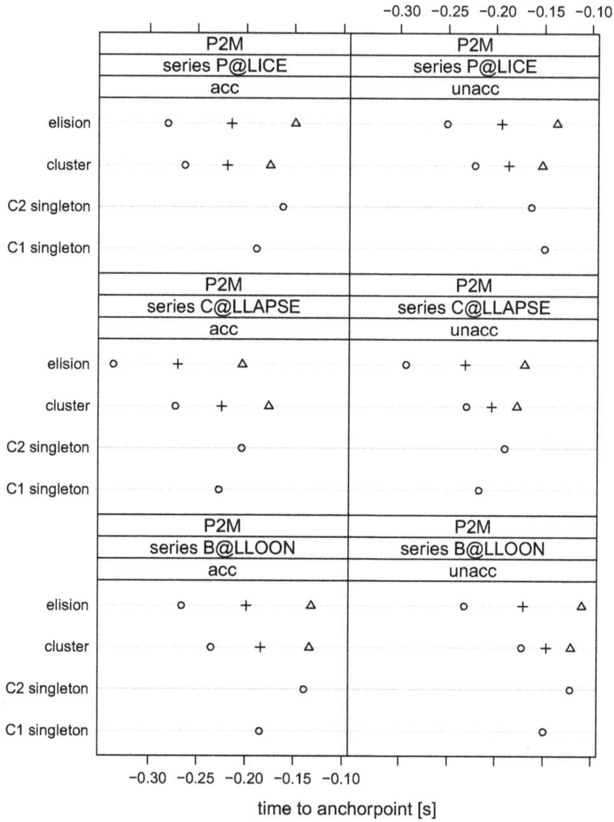

Figure 7. Lags to the rhyme anchor point for onset consonant material, speaker P2M. See Fig. 6 for details.

of any articulatory specification for schwa. The ensemble averages are shown in Figure 8 with the left panels displaying the ensemble averages for speaker P1M, and the right panels those for speaker P2M. The top panels display the *police* series, the middle panel the *balloon* series, and the bottom panel the *collapse* series. For the *balloon* and *police* series, the plotted interval for the bilabial-/l/-sequences is the interval that starts 100 ms prior to the CONSTR ON of the bilabial closing movement and ends 100 ms later than CONSTR OFF of the tongue tip movement. In addition, the interval between CONSTR ON of the bilabial movement and CONSTR OFF of the tongue tip constriction is shown in bold face; the start of the movement is shown by the capital S. Similar intervals were defined for the *collapse*-series accordingly. The main finding is that regardless of the accentuation condition there is evidence for the "targetlessness" of the schwa insofar as the visual inspection of the tongue dorsum trajectories suggests that in most cases their shape is controlled by the consonantal environment and by accentuation. Accented items usually show more extreme turning points towards the stressed vowels than deaccented items, i.e. the trajectories in accented *balloon/bloom* are lower and slightly more retracted than in deaccented items. In contrast, there are no substantial differences between items with a lexical schwa (*police, balloon, collapse*) versus the complex onset condition (*please, bloom, claps*). The fact that trajectory shape is mainly determined by the accentuation seems to confirm earlier results by Browman and Goldstein (1990a) on the targetlessness of schwa in pretonic position and suggests that in most cases the tongue dorsum trajectory in the interval between the two consonants is determined by the surrounding consonants. There are two deviances, both for P1M, the first concerns the *police* series: The unaccented elision condition does not group well with the unaccented cluster condition. Still, this does not result in a regrouping of clusters and elisions. Such a regrouping is observed for the *collapse* series though: Here, speaker P1M indeed has similar trajectory shapes for pretonic syllables and cluster conditions respectively.

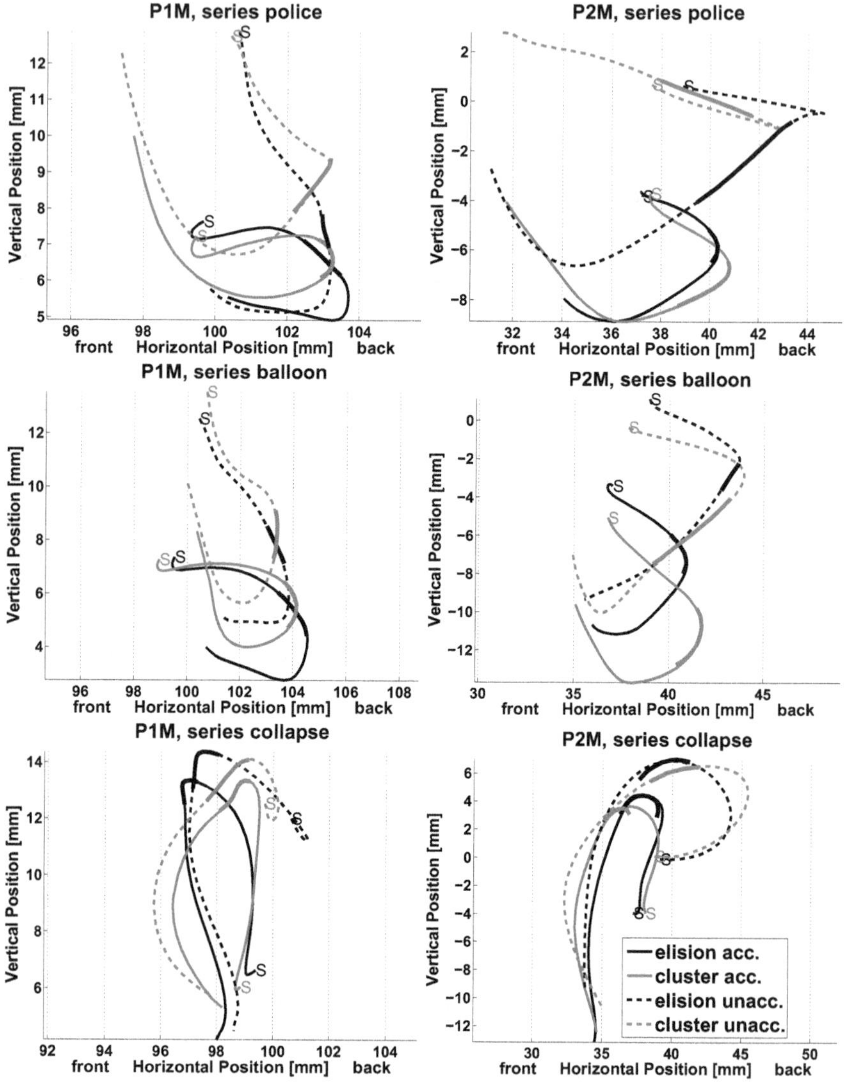

Figure 8. Ensemble Averages of tongue mid sensor for speaker P1M (left panels) and speaker P2M (right panels). The first row shows data for the *police* series, the middle panel contains the data for the *balloon* series. The *collapse* series is shown in the bottom left panels. For further explanation see text.

4 Discussion

This pilot study addressed the behaviour of complex onset clusters and pretonic reduction syllables in English. Results consisted in the findings that pretonic syllables and clusters do not converge into homophones resulting from the prosodic manipulation applied here (see section 2.2). This was shown by patterns of intergestural timing between the consonants, and the analyses of C-centres. Our speakers show a consistent lag between the consonants in the onset cluster. This finding is in agreement with the overlap pattern for 3 French speakers, reported by Hoole et al. (2010), but differs from their German speakers who produced C/l/ clusters with considerable overlap. Nevertheless, the interconsonantal lag for the pretonic case is still longer than the same lag for the cluster case. Results of the spatial patterns are less consistent for our speakers: While one speaker (P2M) consistently lacks a separate target for the pretonic schwa if the tongue dorsum sensor is considered alone, the picture for P1M is less conclusive. However, limitations of the analyses performed so far do not yield a complete picture yet. We plan to extend the analyses to other oral articulatory structures like the lips and the jaw in order to clarify whether there is a target for the schwa or not. In addition, we plan to carry out additional acoustic analysis which could be indicative of the targetlessness of the schwa in the pretonic syllables.

The results presented here are at least in partial agreement with Browman and Goldstein's (1990b) interpretation of the difference between consonant sequences in pretonic schwa syllables and in underlying clusters as a pure difference of temporal coordination. While fully consistent for one of our speakers, the results presented at least do not disconfirm such an analysis for our second participant.

In other words, in the light of the spatial data the scenario in Figure 3, i.e. the representation of the initial CV syllable without vowel seems to be better compatible with the data that we have observed, but is likely to be at odds with most speakers' intuitions. Anyway, this representation bears some similarity with the Schwa-Null-Alternation often assumed as the representation of Schwa in German Phonology (Hall, 1992, Wiese, 1988, both after Hall 2000). According to these views, the underlying representation does not contain the schwa; rather, the surface realization is obtained by epenthesis or, within the framework of Articulatory

Phonology, by a transient schwa generated by a lag between the two consonants.

Rather than furthering these maybe even accidental associations it is in our view more productive to speculate on the reasons for the slight inconsistency of grouping in the spatial patterns that have been observed. The grouping of ensemble averages, which follows by accent condition in the vast majority of cases, is broken for P1M in the *collapse* series. This finding might actually point to a shortcoming of the current experimental design: The current experiment did not make an attempt to more explicitly control speech rate or utilize an increase for eliciting more extreme reductions. In contrast to Davidson (2006) who used speech rate increases for eliciting reductions, Browman and Goldstein (1990a) and the current experiment aimed at using a more natural prosodic variation.

The absolute lag between the two consonants was not affected by accent in a consistent way. Two reasons might be responsible for this: first of all, it has been found that the timing in onset clusters is relatively insensitive to variations in boundary strength (see Byrd and Choi, 2010) as well word stress (see Bombien et al., 2010). This might at least explain why the underlying onset clusters showed very little temporal variation for deaccentuation. The second reason might apply to the pretonic case: as was shown by Turk and White (1999) for American English, deaccentuation affected stressed syllables to a much greater degree than following unstressed syllables. The effect on pretonic syllables was even smaller and also less reliable across speakers. This high degree of speaker specificity might explain why our two speakers showed much smaller effect sizes of deaccentuation in comparison to Browman and Goldstein's (1990a) speaker.

As just suggested, speech rate manipulations might be more effective for further reduction of the pretonic syllable. However, as Davidson (2006) found for American English, only some speakers showed higher elision rates when speaking faster. Furthermore, the study by Jannedy (1994, after Beckman 1996) on German gave evidence for a complete temporal neutralisation only in posttonic syllables, e.g. /n/ in **CC. *Kannen* (i.e. /kˈanən/ → k^hann̩)** approached the same duration as /n/ in *kann* only at the fastest speech rate. Similar results were found by Pompino-Marschall and Janker (1999) whose speakers retained durational differences between *ein* and bisyllabic *einen*. These findings were further corroborated by accompanying perceptual tests. Interestingly, this tendency was less consistent for the pretonic items *beraten* versus *braten* in Jannedy (1994)'s study. Therefore, complete neutralisation of the difference in temporal coordination patterns between underlying onset clusters and consonants in pretonic syllables is not to be expected for Standard German, British English and American English.

Nevertheless, other languages or dialects, such as Bavarian, could well show the same timing in underlying clusters and the Bavarian equivalent of consonant sequences in pretonic syllables. Bavarian is of special interest for this issue because the realization of the prefixes *ge-* and *be-* as in *gsuffa* (Standard German: *gesoffen*, 'drunken' past tense) and *bsuffa* (Standard German: *besoffen*, 'drunk', adjective) is not induced by a change in speaking style or speech rate but a crucial feature of this dialect (see Rowley 1990 for North Bavarian and Wiesinger 1989). The perfect participle /ge-/ is realized as unvoiced unaspirated [k] preceding stems with initial fricatives, nasals, laterals, trills and vowels. Before stops it is completely deleted, e.g. *gekonnt* → *kenna*. Even though this latter restriction seems to imply that phonotactically illegal clusters are avoided, several counterexamples exist, such as *gefragt* → [*kfr*]*ogt*, *geschlagen* → [*kʃl*]*ong*, which do not occur as onsets in simplex words of Bavarian. Furthermore, lexicalized forms can be found frequently, such as *Klump*, derived from *ge+lumpe*, 'junk'. Similar regularities apply to the derivational prefix *be-*. On the one hand, because past tense forms in Bavarian never show a schwa, there may be a stronger tendency towards C-Center timing in these forms than in the standard language. On the other hand, the timing relationships may be sensitive to the morphological complexity of the clusters, so that, for example, lexically given /gl/ clusters may show a stronger C-center effect than /gl/ clusters that emerge from past participle formation. Anyway, Bavarian should allow the possibility of experimentally manipulating morphological complexity, and it therefore would present an interesting test case.

For British English, the difference in C-centre in our and other studies speaks against an integration of the first consonant in e.g. *police* in the stressed syllable and can be viewed as the main property distinguishing the two words from each other since we could not detect a target for the schwa. The absence of the C-centre suggests that these two word forms are distinguished by their coupling graphs, as exemplified in Figures 2 and 3. Further evidence for unsyllabified initial consonants, which are hypothesized not to be in-phase coupled directly to a vowel, were presented for the impure /s/ in Italian by Hermes et al. (2008), Moroccan Arabic by Shaw et al. (2009), and for Tashlhiyt Berber by Goldstein et al. (2010).

However, the C-centre analyzes presented in Figures 6 and 7 of the current study might have suffered from problems to generate test materials with well-defined anchor points. For example the problem in the *police* series is that the vowel in *please* may be inherently longer than in *police*, related to the voiced vs. voiceless fricative in the coda (see Chen, 1970). This effect might have shifted the whole cluster further to the left than expected. However, this does not explain the short durations in *lease*, so this effect might not ultimately be separable from the effects of polysyllabic shortening that were discussed in 3.1.2. Another potentially interfering effect depending on the choice of the anchor consonant is the contrast between *balloon* versus *bloom*, but here it remains unclear how this could have affected the results. The choice of the anchor consonant cannot be responsible for the differences in alignment between *boon* and *loon*. Still, in a future version of the corpus it would advisable to record items like *boom* and *loom* in addition. Apart from these more specific effects of corpus design, the paper by Goldstein et al. (2010) addresses the possibility that there are examples in which the same syllable structure is associated with different timing patterns depending on factors like place of articulation, manner or language studied. Rather than offering an extension of the task dynamic model that could account for deviations of such a constant C-centre, the analysis focused on whether there is the predicted left-shift of the first onset consonant and a simultaneous right shift of the second onset consonant C_2. A gross examination of our data does show a lack of right-shift for C_2 but the left shift for C_1 and the longer lag between the two consonants are extremely consistent and speak for fundamentally different timing constellations depending on syllable structure and onset complexity.

5 Acknowledgement

This research was funded by grants to the EPSRC (EP/E01609X/1, EP/-E016359/1), the NIH (NIDCD DC008780) and the German Research Council (HO3271/3-2). We also wish to thank Pascal Perrier and Susanne Fuchs for invaluable comments on a draft version of the paper.

References

Beckman, M. (1996). When is a syllable not a syllable? In Otake, T. and Cutler, A., editors, *Phonological structure and language processing: cross-linguistic studies*, pages 111–146. Mouton de Gruyter, Berlin.

Bombien, L., Mooshammer, C., Hoole, P., and Kühnert, B. (2010). Prosodic and segmental effects on EPG contact patterns of word-initial German clusters. *Journal of Phonetics*.

Browman, C. and Goldstein, L. (1990a). Gestural specification using dynamically-defined articulatory structures. *Journal of Phonetics*, 18:299–320.

Browman, C. and Goldstein, L. (1990b). Tiers in articulatory phonology, with some implications for casual speech. In Kingston, J. and Beckman, M. E., editors, *Papers in Laboratory Phonology I: Between the Grammar and Physics of Speech*, pages 341–376. Cambridge, Cambridge, UK.

Browman, C. and Goldstein, L. (1994). "Targetless" schwa: an articulatory analysis. In Docherty, G. and Ladd, D., editors, *Papers in Laboratory Phonology II: Gesture, Segment, Prosody*, pages 26–56. Cambridge University Press: Cambridge.

Browman, C. P. and Goldstein, L. M. (2000). Competing constraints on intergestural coordination and self-organization of phonological structures. *Les Cahiers de l'ICP, Bulletin de la Communication Parlée*, 5:25–34.

Byrd, D. (1996). A phase window framework for articulatory timing. *Phonology*, 13:139–169.

Byrd, D. and Choi, S. (2010). At the juncture of prosody, phonology, and phonetics – the interaction of phrasal and syllable structure in shaping the timing of consonant gestures. In Fougeron, C., Kühnert, B., d'Imperio, M., and Vallée, N., editors, *Papers in Laboratory Phonology 10: Variation, Detail and Representation*. Mouton de Gruyter.

Chen, M. (1970). Vowel length variation as a function of the variety of the consonant environment. *Phonetica*, 22:129–159.

Davidson, L. (2006). Schwa elision in fast speech: segmental deletion or gestural overlap? *Phonetica*, 63:79–112.

Goldstein, L., Nam, H., Saltzman, E., and Chitoran, I. (2010). Coupled oscillator planning model of speech timing and syllable structure. In Fant, G., Fujisaki, H., and Shen, J., editors, *Frontiers in Phonetics and Speech Science, Festschrift for Wu Zongji*, pages 239–250. Commercial Press, Beijing.

Haken, H., Kelso, J., and Bunz, H. (1985). A theoretical model of phase transitions in human hand movements. *Biological Cybernetics*, 51:347–356.

Hall, T. (2000). *Phonologie. Eine Einführung*. Berlin, New York: De Gruyter.

Hall, T. A. (1992). *Syllable structure and syllable-related processes in German*. Linguistische Arbeiten 276. Niemeyer-Varlag, Tübingen.

Hermes, A., Grice, M., Mücke, D., and Niemann, H. (2008). Articulatory indicators of syllable liason in word initial consonant clusters in Italian. In *Proceedings of the 8th International Seminar on Speech Production*, pages 433–436.

Honorof, D. and Browman, C. (1995). The centre or edge: how are consonant clusters organised with respect to the vowel? In Elenius, K. and Branderud, P., editors, *Proceedings of the XIIIth International Congress of Phonetic Sciences*, pages 552–555.

Hoole, P., Bombien, L., Kühnert, B., and Mooshammer, C. (2010). Intrinsic and prosodic effects on articulatory coordination in initial consonant clusters. In Fant, G., Fujisaki, H., and Shen, J., editors, *Frontiers in Phonetics and Speech Science, Festschrift for Wu Zongji*, pages 281–291. Commercial Press, Beijing.

Hoole, P. and Zierdt, A. (2010). Five-dimensional articulography. In Maassen, B. and van Lieshout, P., editors, *Speech Motor Control: New developments in basic and applied research*, pages 331–349. Oxford University Press, Oxford, U.K.

Hoole, P., Zierdt, A., and Geng, C. (2003). Beyond 2D in articulatory data acquisition and analysis. In *Proceedings of the 15th International Congress of Phonetic Sciences*, pages 265–268.

Hooper, J. (1978). Constrains on schwa-deletion in american english. In Fisiak, J., editor, *Recent Developments in Historical Linguisitics.*, pages 193–207. The Hague: Mouton.

Jannedy, S. (1994). Rate effects on german unstressed syllables. *Working Papers in Linguistics, Ohio State University*, 44:105–124.

Kaisse, E. (1985). *Connected Speech: The Interaction of Syntax and Phonology*. San Diego: Academic Press.

Krakow, R. A. (1999). Physiological organization of syllables: a review. *Journal of Phonetics*, 27:23–54.

Nam, H. and Saltzman, E. (2003). A competitive, coupled oscillator model of syllable structure. In Solé, M.-J., Recasens, D., and Romero, J., editors, *Proceedings of the 15th International Congress of Phonetic Sciences*, pages 2253–2256, Barcelona. Futurgrafic.

Pompino-Marschall, B. and Janker, P. M. (1999). Production and perception of syllabic [n] in German. In *Proceedings of the 14th International Congress of Phonetic Sciences (San Francisco)*.

Rowley, A. (1990). North Bavarian. In Russ, C., editor, *The Dialects of Modern German.*, pages 417–437. Routledge, London.

Saltzman, E., Nam, H., and Goldstein, L. (sub.). Intergestural timing in speech production: the role of graph structure.

Saltzman, E., Nam, H., Krivokapic, J., and Goldstein, L. (2008). A task-dynamic toolkit for modeling the effects of prosodic structure on articulation. In Barbosa, P. A., Madureira, S., and Reis, C., editors, *Proceedings of the Speech Prosody 2008*, pages 175–184.

Shaw, J., Gafos, I. A., Hoole, P., and Zeroual, C. (2009). Syllabification in Moroccan Arabic: evidence from temporal stability in articulation. *Phonology (Yearbook)*, 26:187–215.

Smorodinsky, I. (2002). *Schwas with and without active gestural control.* PhD thesis, Yale University.

Turk, A. and Shattuck-Hufnagel, S. (2000). Word-boundary-related durational patterns in English. *Journal of Phonetics*, 28:397–440.

Turk, E. A. and White, L. (1999). Structural influences on accentual lengthening in English. *Journal of Phonetics*, 27:171–206.

Wiese, R. (1988). *Silbische und lexikalische Phonologie.* Linguistische Arbeiten 211. Niemeyer, Tübingen.

Wiesinger, P. (1989). *Die Flexionsmorphologie des Verbums im Bairischen.* Verlag der Österreichischen Akademie der Wissenschaften.

Velar and Glottal Activity in Icelandic*

Philip Hoole
Lasse Bombien

Abstract: Transillumination data was used to analyze laryngeal-oral coordination in Icelandic pre-aspirated plosives and groups of voiceless nasal plus plosive (together with comparison items with unaspirated plosive, and voiced nasal plus plosive). Analysis focussed firstly on whether pre-aspirated plosives are better regarded not as a counterpart to familiar (post)-aspirated plosives but rather as a sequence of /h/+plosive, and secondly on the phonemic status of voiceless nasals, given the existence of apparent minimal pairs of voiceless vs. voiced nasal followed by plosive (for one of the three subjects photoelectric data on velar movement supplemented the laryngeal data). Little evidence was found for regarding pre-aspirated plosives as /h/+plosive. This, in turn, makes it possible to closely link pre-aspirated plosives and voiceless nasals within a coarticulatory framework. The voiceless nasals are best regarded as not having phonemic status but rather as emerging from coarticulation with a following pre-aspirated plosive, thus forming a counterpart to the coarticulatory voicelessness of sonorants in sequences such as /pl/ in languages with post-aspirated plosives.

* The first author would like to thank Bernd Pompino-Marschall for awakening his interest in the topic of articulatory coordination in general, and, in particular, for recruiting the main subject. Both authors would like to thank him for the extensive opportunities they have enjoyed to acquire laryngeal fiberoptic and transillumination data at the phonetics lab of Zentrum für Allgemeine Sprachwissenschaft, Berlin. An acknowledgement is also in order to the Icelandic volcano Eyjafjallajökull (['ɛɪjaˌfjatlaˌjœkʏtl̥]) for raising public awareness of devoicing of sonorants, and, by disrupting air-traffic, for giving the first author the enforced leisure necessary to finalize the manuscript. Thanks also to Christine Mooshammer and an anonymous reviewer for constructive comments.

1 Introduction[1]

In 1958 Haugen declared that "there is probably little to be added of purely phonetic detail" to the description of Icelandic. Undeterred by this, a number of investigators have since then looked closely at various aspects of Icelandic phonetics (e.g. Pétursson, 1972, 1973a, 1975, 1976; Garnes, 1973; Löfqvist and Yoshioka, 1980). Indeed, as the latter have pointed out, Icelandic provides plenty of scope for investigations of the temporal organization of speech. Their work concentrated on glottal activity, including pre-aspirated plosives, which is a main focus of interest here. A further noteworthy aspect of Icelandic is the existence of voiceless nasals (see Pétursson, 1973b, for a phonological analysis), which thus involve the coordination of labial or lingual, velar and glottal gestures.

In this work we will consider velar and glottal activity in pre-aspirated plosives and voiceless nasals as part of the more general aim of using phonetic analysis to throw light on phonological problems. We will attempt to show that pre-aspirated plosives and voiceless nasals are more closely related than has often been assumed to be the case, particularly when these sounds are viewed from the perspective of coarticulatory processes. At this point the phonetic and phonological background to these sounds must be discussed in greater detail and the hypotheses forming the backbone of the experimental investigations expounded more fully. Our debt to Pétursson's work will be clear, although we take issue with him on a number of points.

1 The work presented here has had a convoluted history: A preliminary version appeared many years ago as a conference presentation in Hoole (1987). A longer version was then prepared, but never submitted for publication. It eventually formed the appendix to an unpublished habilitation thesis on laryngeal articulation (Hoole, 2006a). The present version now supplements the single original speaker with more recent laryngeal data for two additional speakers (details in Bombien (2006)). Apart from these new data the introductory and results sections of the present paper still reflect the way in which the issues were formulated for the original paper. The results, the underlying questions, and the preliminary discussion in Section 4 are placed in the perspective of more recent literature in the concluding Section 5 ("General Discussion")

1.1 Pre-aspirated plosives

Let us start with the pre-aspirated plosives. Phonetically, it is firmly established that they are produced with glottal abduction starting well before implosion of the plosive itself (by implosion we mean the time-point at the onset of consonantal closure at which a sharp rise in intra-oral air-pressure begins). In fact, implosion corresponds roughly to the time at which peak glottal opening (PGO) occurs. A hardy annual in the field of Icelandic phonology has been the question of quantity, since Icelandic possesses quite a rich pattern of contrasting vowel and consonant durations. Here we will be referring to it only in passing. It is of relevance to the pre-aspirated plosives, however, since these sounds have traditionally been described as long, the voiceless unaspirated as short, e.g. 'seppi' (pre-aspirated) vs. 'sepi' (unaspirated). Previous experimental evidence tends to show (Garnes, 1973) that there is not much to choose between these sounds as far as length of the *occlusion* is concerned (in fact, the occlusion for the pre-aspirated stop may even be shorter than for the unaspirated case; Pétursson (1972)).

Pre-aspirated plosives occur only word-medially, e.g. 'seppi', and finally, e.g. 'löpp'. (leg) In combination with other consonants they occur only before /l/ and /n/, e.g. 'epli'(apple), 'opna' (open).

Pétursson adduces a number of arguments aiming to show that the pre-aspirated plosives are better regarded as combinations of /h/ + Plosive (abbreviated to 'P' below):

a) The duration of prevocalic /h/ and the pre-aspiration phase are approximately the same.
b) The duration of pre-aspiration and occlusion are much the same. Put another way, pre-aspiration is proportionately very long compared with post-aspiration in Icelandic or other languages. Pétursson seems to feel awkward about the idea that an aspiration phase can be as long as the occlusion to which it 'belongs'. He also seems to expect pre-aspiration, if such it is, to be a kind of mirror-image of post-aspiration. It is difficult to see the force of this argument, since there may be psycho-acoustic reasons why aspiration linked to vowel offset needs to be longer for perceptual saliency than aspiration linked to vowel onset.

c) He observed a slight lowering of the velum both for instances of /h/ and pre-aspiration in his cineradiographic investigations.
d) The posited consonantal groups /h/ + P have a similar temporal structure to other groups of C + P.

While Pétursson was perfectly aware of the restricted number of examples on which his analysis was based, and forgetting for a moment the reservations already stated, the analysis as a whole seems quite plausible. In particular it has the merit of fitting in with the prediction that a plosive following a voiceless consonant is unaspirated.
However, we think it will be possible to show, on the basis of our own data, that none of the arguments taken individually really hold water. This will be the first step in support of the hypothesis regarding voiceless nasals to which we will now turn.

1.2 The voiceless nasals

Icelandic is certainly remarkable for the large number of phonetically identifiable nasals (see Pétursson, 1973b, for a review), generally being considered to include four voiced ([m, n, ŋ, ɲ]), and the corresponding four voiceless nasals (as well as four constrictives). (We leave aside the palatal and velars here, as their phonemic status is debatable). The occurrence of voiceless nasals is not the same in all parts of Iceland, although their distribution is severely restricted everywhere. In the North they occur only in word final position following another voiceless consonant, e.g. 'lasm' [lasm̥] (*friend*), and would appear to be allophones of the corresponding voiced nasals since they become voiced again if followed by another voiced sound, e.g. 'vatn' (*water*) [va^{h}tn̥#] vs. 'vatni' (dat. sing.) [va^{h}tnɪ#].
In the South the same situation obtains; however in addition voiceless nasals can occur before /p, t, k/ following a short vowel (for details again see Pétursson). They are thus restricted to positions in which the pre-aspirated plosives also occur. Apparent examples of minimal pairs contrasting voiced and voiceless nasals are easy enough to find in this position, e.g. 'dempi' [dɛm̥pɪ] vs. 'dembi' [dɛmpɪ], so there is a prima facie case for regarding the voiceless nasals as phonemes in Southern Icelandic. In the North the situation is different since 'dempi' etc. is realized as [dɛmp^{h}ɪ] - contrasting through the post-aspiration with

'dembi' ([dɛmpi]).[2] The only experimental investigation, to our knowledge, which has examined voiced and voiceless nasals in Southern Icelandic is also due to Pétursson (1975). His main findings were that in such minimal pairs:

a) Voiceless nasals are longer than voiced.
b) The difference in plosive duration following voiceless vs. voiced nasals is very small (any tendency was in the direction of shorter plosives after voiceless nasals).
c) Vowels preceding the different nasals are essentially the same length.
d) There was no clear difference in velar opening.

Pétursson was unable to give any measurements of the speed of the velar gesture, but he hypothesized that velar raising would be faster in the voiceless nasals. He takes the view that since the plosives in pairs such as 'dempi/dembi' are not reliably different in length, and since they are voiceless in both cases, the nasals are the bearers of the phonological contrast between such pairs and therefore belong to different phonemes.[3]

We will be attempting to use experimental evidence to show that it is more elegant to regard the voiceless nasals as normal nasals coarticulated with pre-aspirated plosives.

This idea is not new. Haugen took the view that both *"pre- and post-aspiration are components of fortis stops"*, and that the voiceless continuants (i.e. including nasals) are in complementary distribution with the voiced, since *"in the position before aspirated* [i.e. also pre-aspirated (authors' note)] *stops voicelessness is closely correlated to the aspiration of the stops and in general appears to be determined by it"* (1958, p. 73). The position of the aspiration would be stated in an allophonic rule.

The need for an allophonic rule of this kind has been a source of disquiet to some, e.g. Werner (1963), who plumps for the phonemicity of voiced and voiceless nasals in Faroese where a somewhat similar situation applies.

It is perhaps unfortunate that Haugen could not phrase his explanation in terms of coarticulation since Pétursson has consistently rejected his

2 Pre-aspiration itself does also occur in Northern Icelandic in the words such as 'seppi' given in the previous section.

3 The more recent paper of Jessen and Pétursson (1998) also comes to the conclusion that there are no consistent differences in duration of the plosive following the different nasals. This paper is considered in more detail below in the General Discussion.

point of view, possibly as a result of a misunderstanding: *"Haugens Argumente sind wertlos, weil es aus physiologischen Gründen weder einen aspirierten noch einen stimmhaften Verschlusslaut nach stimmlosem Nasal geben kann"* (1975, p. 653)[4]. This is the more curious since Pétursson (1973a) has himself given a plausible account in coarticulatory terms of the genesis of pre-aspirates and voiceless nasals, in which the appearance of the two groups of sounds is closely linked, and attributed to the same process, namely a shift in the timing of a ballistic devoicing gesture.

However, Pétursson was already convinced for the reasons given above that pre-aspirates are phonemically /h/+P, and on this basis it is only consistent to regard the voiceless nasals as phonemes as well.

As already intimated at the beginning of the introduction, we believe that in fact it will be possible to argue that the most consistent picture of these sounds emerges if this coarticulatory perspective is retained for the synchronic analysis as well.

In short, the line of argument to be followed below is as follows:

First, the pre-aspirates must be examined. If no compelling reason is found for regarding them as sequences of /h/+plosive, then viewing voiceless nasals as a consequence of coarticulation with a following pre-aspirated plosive becomes a possible scenario. For the scenario to be not just possible but plausible we then need to show similarity in the glottal behaviour of the two classes of sounds. In addition, further articulatory and acoustic comparison of voiceless and voiced nasals also needs to be compatible with regarding them as allophones of the same phoneme.

2 Material, method, subjects

The recordings were carried out in two parts. The first part consisted of recordings of laryngeal movement, velar movement, and intraoral airpressure for a single subject (S1). These will be referred to as the main recordings. The second part consisted of recordings of laryngeal movement for a subset of the material for two additional subjects (S2 and S3). These will be referred to as supplementary recordings.

4 "Haugen's arguments have no value, because for physiological reasons it is not possible to have either an aspirated or voiced occlusive following a voiceless nasal".

2.1 Main recordings

A male speaker of Southern Icelandic ('linmæli') acted as subject. He had been studying in Germany for four years but visited Iceland regularly and was in constant contact with fellow Icelanders in Germany. The speech material was chosen to permit contrast of pre-aspirated plosives, unaspirated plosives, voiceless nasal plus plosive and voiced nasal plus plosive in as homogeneous an environment as possible. This led to the following list of two groups of four words each, the sounds of interest all being in medial, post-stress position.

hitti	hɪ^{h}tɪ	pre-asp	*meet* (1 sg. pret)
hiti	hɪ:tɪ	unasp	*heat* (nom. Sg. m)
henti	hɛn̥tɪ	voiceless N	*throw away* (1 sg. pret)
hendi	hɛntɪ	voiced N	*hand* (dat. Sg. f)

seppi	sɛ^{h}pɪ	pre-asp	*dog* (name)
sepi	sɛ:pɪ	unasp	*rag*
dempi	dɛm̥pɪ	voiceless N	*dampen* (1. Sg. pres. Conj.)
dembi	dɛmpɪ	voiced N	*throw* (1 sg pres conj.)

One additional word each for the pre-aspirate and voiceless nasal case were also included ('sempinn' is lexically somewhat marginal):

hetta	hɛ^{h}ta	pre-asp	*hood*
sempinn	sɛm̥pɪn	voiceless N	*base, common*

The long vowels preceding the unaspirated plosives are generally somewhat diphthongized.
Back vowels and consonants were excluded from the material since they can cause artefacts in the photoelectroglottographic signal. In fact, for the purposes of the experiment this is not a very grave restriction since velar/palatal voiceless nasals are much rarer than their bilabial and alveolar counterparts. A further methodological word of warning is in order here: movement of the velum could also lead to artefacts in the PGG signal for the voiceless nasals, however the risk seemed worth taking.
This list of 10 words was subjected to six different randomizations thus dividing the material into six blocks. To reduce list effects some dummy

items were inserted at the beginning and end of each block. The words were embedded in the sentence frame "Ég segi ____ þá" (" *I say* ____ *then*").

The following procedure was followed for the recordings: Glottal activity was assessed using the transillumination technique (F-J Electronics' photoelectroglottograph), the light source being applied between the thyroid and cricoid cartilages, and the light passing through the glottis being picked up by a catheter-mounted phototransistor inserted nasally into the pharynx. Here the devoicing gesture was of principal interest, and for this the method is considered quite reliable (Hutters, 1976; Löfqvist and Yoshioka, 1980), particularly for information on the timing of the gesture, while amplitude information should be interpreted with rather more caution.

Velar activity was monitored using the fiberoptic method developed by Künzel (1979). A fiberoptic bundle containing a light guide and photo transistor is inserted into the nasal cavity. The phototransistor picks up the light reflected from the upper surface of the velum. The relationship between velar height and amount of light reflected is considered to be basically linear (Künzel, 1979). Since the velograph also uses the photoelectroglottograph as light source and since we only had one instrument available velar and glottal activity had to be recorded separately. (Had two instruments been available it is still questionable whether simultaneous recording would have been possible because of interference between the light sources and catheters.) To ensure that all recordings were spoken at roughly the same rate the first recording was recorded on tape, and pauses were inserted. This tape was then played back to the subject over earphones in subsequent recordings, and he was asked to speak in the pause following the model. A total of three recordings was made. In each, the audio signal and the physiological signal were digitized and stored on magnetic tape on-line, the audio signal at a sample rate of 10 kHz, the physiological one at 5 kHz. The physiological signals were the photoelectroglottgram in the first recording, the velogram in the second and the intra-oral air-pressure in the third. The latter was registered via a Hanson Manometer and catheter also inserted through the nose into the pharynx. This last recording was used to fill in some of the details of plosive articulation and as a cross-check on the segmentation methods used in the first two. Following storage, a graphically-assisted segmentation program was used to measure the following parameters (for the words in the 'basic' list):

1. Length of the vowel preceding the consonant or consonant group
2. Length of the nasal or length of pre-aspiration, based on the audio signal
3. Length of the occlusion for the plosive
4. Size of PGO (peak glottal opening) and its position relative to onset and offset of the preceding vowel
5. Maximum speed of glottal opening and its position
6. Maximum speed of glottal closing and its position
7. Maximum speed of velar lowering
8. Maximum speed of velar raising
9. Velar excursion
10. Interval between moment of maximum speed of glottal opening and closing
11. Interval between moment of maximum speed of velar lowering and raising.

For calculation of the parameters based on the physiological signals (i.e. parameters 4-11 in the above list) the raw signals were first smoothed and, for the sub-set based on velocities (i.e. parameters 5-8, 10, 11), velocities were then determined by successive subtractions over 10 ms. steps. As further timing parameters, interest was also attached to determination of the onset of velar lowering and glottal abduction. For the latter, we have shown that in German the time-point at which glottal abduction starts is the same for plosives and fricatives if measured from onset of the preceding vowel. We were curious to see whether similar relationships obtain for other classes of sounds, and in other languages (see Hoole et al., 1984). However, these measurements presented some difficulties for reasons to be outlined in the results below (in section 3.2.2 for glottal movements; in section 3.2.3 for velar movements). From the air-pressure curves only peak air-pressure in the occlusions was determined.

2.2 Supplementary recordings

These recordings were carried out nearly 20 years after the main recordings and used a different arrangement of the transillumination technique for capturing laryngeal movements. Specifically, the larynx was filmed (video) using an Olympus ENF-P3 fiberscope.[5] The endoscopic light-source simultaneously provided the light for the transillumination signal, which was registered by means of phototransistors attached externally to the neck below the level of the glottis. Details of this technique, together with further discussion of methodological issues, can be found in Hoole (1999b, 2006b).

Two subjects (S2 and S3) recorded a corpus for the investigation of Icelandic sonorants that is presented in detail in Bombien (2006). It included four items that overlapped with the corpus of the main recordings, namely 'hitti', 'hiti', 'henti' and 'hendi',i.e. one item for each of the four consonant categories of interest. For both speakers 8-10 repetitions of these items were available for analysis. These data will be used to supplement the data from S1 for the analysis of acoustically based segment durations (principally section 3.1) and laryngeal kinematics (section 3.2.1 and 3.2.2).

3 Results

3.1 Basic segment durations

3.1.1 Main recordings

We will begin presentation of the results by mentioning some of the grosser aspects of the temporal organisation of the material investigated. By this are meant effects that are still apparent when the results of all three recordings for S1 are merged. This will then provide a framework for more precise discussion of the physiological parameters. The words will be treated as consisting of a maximum of three basic segments: 1. The vowel preceding the consonantal group; 2. The nasal or pre-aspiration section; 3. The occlusion phase of the plosive. Figure 1 shows the results for S1 in graphical form, averaging over all three recordings and over all word forms within each linguistic category. Table 1 shows a breakdown for each word form in the corpus and also includes the supplementary data from S2 and S3. On the basis of vowel length the

5 These recordings were carried out at ZAS, Berlin, with the kind assistance of Dr. Klaus Dahlmeier.

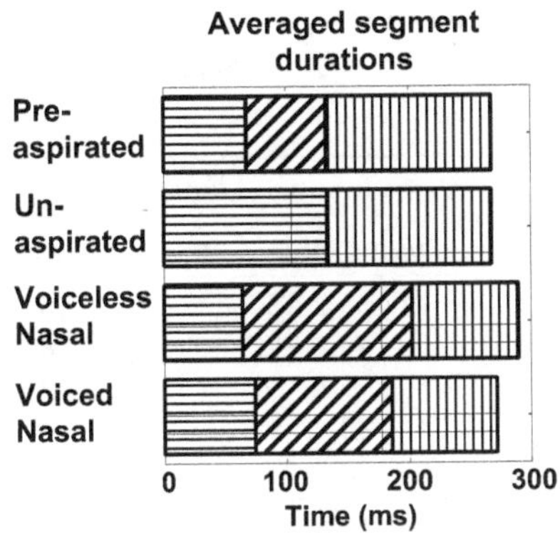

Figure 1. Average duration ofs the three basic segments for each of the main linguistic categories. Horizontal hatching: Vowel; Diagonal hatching: Pre-aspiration or Nasal (absent for the unaspirated category); Vertical hatching: Plosive occlusion.

material fell into two groups, one group consisting only of sepi, and hiti, in which the (diphthongized) vowel was 120-140 ms in length (segment 2 being completely lacking here of course) and a second group containing all other words, in which the length of the vowel was roughly 60-85 ms. As far as segment 2 is concerned, the length of pre-aspiration was clearly shorter than that of the nasals - 50-70 ms vs. 110-150 ms. Within the nasals the voiceless sounds tended to be longer than the voiced counterparts (see below for more precise evaluation). The length of segment 3, the plosive occlusion, tended to counterbalance the length of segment 2 with much shorter plosives following the nasals than in the pre-aspirated or unaspirated conditions - ca. 80 ms vs. ca. 120-140 ms.

3.1.2 Supplementary recordings

The results of S2 and S3, given in Table 1, are comparable to those of S1 in all the following respects: 1. relative length of pre-aspiration and nasal segments, i.e. the pre-aspiration (in 'hitti') is clearly shorter than the nasal segments (in 'henti' and 'hendi'); 2. the nasal segment is longer in the voiceless than voiced nasals; 3. the plosive occlusion durations are shorter in the words with nasals than in the pre-aspirated and unaspirated category. The only substantial difference from the temporal pat-

Table 1. Mean (in bold face) and sd of segment durations (in ms), For main subject (S1) averaged over all three reordings (n=18). For supplementary subjects (S2, S3), n=8-10.

			Duration in (ms)		
Word	Categ.	S	vowel	nasal/preasp.	occlusion
seppi	Pre-	1	**59** ± 5.7	**76** ± 10.0	**123** ± 14.9
hetta	asp.	1	**70** ± 7.2	**67** ± 8.4	**136** ± 15.9
hitti		1	**75** ± 9.0	**51** ± 12.5	**146** ± 20.7
hitti		2	**80** ± 9.8	**17** ± 4.8	**73** ± 15.4
hitti		3	**85** ± 10.3	**44** ± 20.0	**115** ± 6.3
sepi	Un-	1	**125** ± 14.4		**134** ± 16.1
hiti	asp.	1	**142** ± 14.5		**134** ± 16.4
hiti		2	**86** ± 8.2		**71** ± 5.3
hiti		3	**88** ± 16.3		**131** ± 7.8
dempi	Voice-	1	**68** ± 4.4	**143** ± 10.5	**87** ± 15.3
sempinn	less	1	**62** ± 4.5	**130** ± 10.6	**83** ± 15.1
henti	Nasal	1	**63** ± 10.4	**141** ± 13.5	**92** ± 11.2
henti		2	**57** ± 3.1	**82** ± 8.2	**42** ± 5.5
henti		3	**57** ± 8.0	**116** ± 19.0	**83** ± 11.1
dembi	Voiced	1	**86** ± 5.2	**108** ± 12.2	**79** ± 20.8
hendi	Nasal	1	**63** ± 6.0	**115** ± 11.7	**92** ± 12.7
hendi		2	**50** ± 10.5	**65** ± 10.2	**55** ± 11.4
hendi		3	**54** ± 12.5	**78** ± 11.7	**103** ± 18.8

terns of S1 involves a less central concern of the present investigation, namely the fact that the newer subjects show no evidence of longer vowels in unaspirated 'hiti'. A further less striking difference is that the new subjects show rather shorter vowels for words with nasals than those without. The main difference between the new subjects is that S2 has shorter occlusion (and also pre-aspiration) durations than S3, despite having very similar vowel durations.

3.2 Glottal and velar activity in detail

Continuing on from the overview of the temporal structure of the utterances given in the previous section we will now discuss in detail the relevant laryngeal and velar kinematics. Figures 2 and 3 show ensemble averages for the glottal and velar signals, together with the audio amplitude envelope, of 8 of the 10 words examined for S1 (i.e. two words for each of the four linguistic categories). Table 2 gives the magnitude of peak glottal opening for S2 and S3. These serve to indicate that all three subjects agreed in the gross features of laryngeal behaviour, i.e. no glottal opening for the voiced nasal category, weak abduction for the unaspirated, and substantial abduction for the pre-aspirated and voiceless nasals. Whether the latter two categories nevertheless differ in their laryngeal kinematics will be considered in detail below.

Table 2. Mean peak glottal opening amplitude for the supplementary subjects (n=9)

	Mean Peak Glottal Opening in Volt	
Word	S2	S3
hitti	1.91	1.85
hiti	0.25	0.53
henti	1.94	2.01
hendi	-0.01	-0.02

Quantitative analysis for S1 was supported, where appropriate, by 2 x 2 analyses of variance carried out on the relevant pairs from the basic word list. In order to counter to some extent such problems as zero drift and variations in gain in the physiological signals the raw data were normalized by converting the data in each block of repetitions to zero mean and unit standard deviation. For S2 and S3 (where only glottal kinematics are relevant) there was an insufficient range of material in the word-medial position for the kind of normalization just mentioned to be appropriate. Accordingly, statistical testing was based on Wilcoxon signed rank tests with word pairs (e.g. a pre-aspirated and a voiceless nasal pair) matched by block (repetition number). This non-parametric procedure (apart from being insensitive to outliers in general) can be assumed to be relatively insensitive to changes in the gain in the transillumination signal, caused, for example, by changes in the position of the fiberscope, over the course of the recording (such changes were indeed clearly present). We turn first to the results bearing on the phonological analysis of the pre-aspirates and nasals.

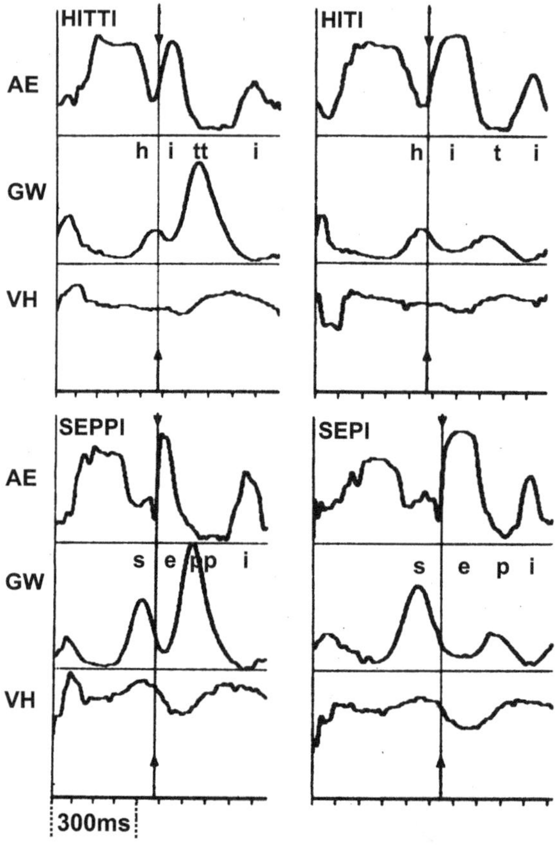

Figure 2. Ensemble averages for pre-aspirated and unaspirated consonants of S1. From top to bottom: Audio Envelope (AE); Glottal Width (GW) from the photoglottographic signal; Velar Height (VH) from the velograph signal. Line-up point (line with arrow) at onset of vowel preceding target consonant. Lower-case transliteration in GW panels indicates rough alignment of segments. No units are shown for the glottal and velar movement signals because the signals from the phototransistors cannot be calibrated. However, across Figures 2 and 3 all sub-panels for a given signal are shown with the same scaling.

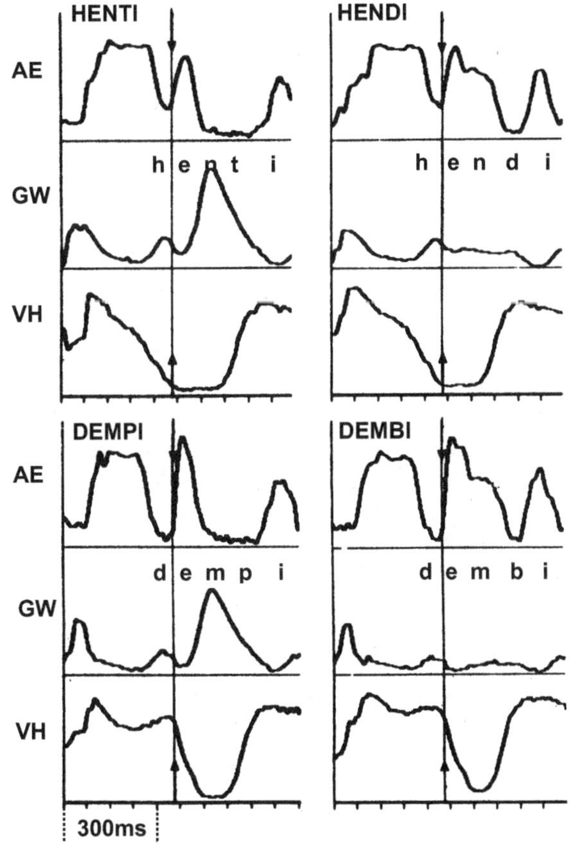

Figure 3. Ensemble averages for voiceless and voiced nasals of S1. Other details as in Figure 2.

3.2.1 Pre-aspiration or /h/

Regarding the duration of pre-aspiration, it has already been pointed out that the length of pre-aspiration and the length of nasals preceding the plosive is quite different and that, in general, sequences of nasal plus plosive are structured differently from sequences (if this is the right word) of pre-aspiration plus plosive. Furthermore, the length of pre-aspiration, even for subjects S1 and S2 with the longest pre-aspiration segments, was never anywhere near as long as the subsequent occlusion (see Table 1). Thus in Pétursson's terms the results for these speakers do not offer much support for his hypothesis.

The main point in this subsection is whether the relevant glottal activity suggests a close connection between pre-aspiration and /h/. The material gives a wealth of examples of /h/ in prevocalic, word-initial, pre-stress position. Comparing in particular glottal activity for /h/ and for the occlusive in 'hitti' for S1 in Figure 2 it is quite clear that activity for /h/ is rather restrained compared with the pre-aspirates (the same applies to 'hetta', which is not shown in the ensemble averages; note also the clearly smaller opening for /h/ than for the voiceless nasal in 'henti' in Figure 3). The differences are large enough to make any non-linearities in the PGG signal negligible. The differences are the more striking since the pre-stress position for /h/ might have been expected to support a more vigorous glottal gesture.

Of the supplementary speakers, the results for S3 were very similar to those of S1: the magnitude of glottal opening was significantly larger for the pre-aspirate of 'hitti' than the initial /h/ ($p<0.01$). For S2 the pre-aspirate had only a marginally larger opening, and this did not approach significance ($p>0.6$). For both these speakers, just as for S1, the glottal opening for the voiceless nasal was significantly larger than the initial /h/ ($p<0.05$ for S2, $p<0.01$ for S3). We will see below that there is no strong evidence for differences in the glottal gesture of the pre-aspirates and the voiceless nasals. The present section thus indicates overall more vigorous glottal abduction for these medial consonantal articulations than for initial /h/.[6] Pétursson considers the extensive ges-

6 In view of the equivocal result for S2 (a significant difference from /h/ for voiceless nasals but not pre-aspirates) and the fact that in the next section he showed no trace of a difference between glottal activity for the pre-aspirates and voiceless nasals, we re-ran

ture for pre-aspirates to be essentially similar to that of other combinations of two voiceless consonants, and this as support for the position that two consonants are in fact present here. What is the basis for deciding which aspect should carry more weight? The similarity in gesture for supposed two-consonant-clusters, or the dissimilarity beween the gesture for pre-vocalic and pre-consonantal /h/? We would suggest that arguments based on similarities or dissimilarities do not take us very far - at least if the aerodynamic and physiological setting in which the language's phonological contrasts have to be produced is not taken into account. The following remarks could be made here: It is conceivable that a larger amplitude of glottal opening is necessary for audible aspiration when this is to be superimposed on a closing movement of the vocal tract (i.e.pre-aspiration) than on an opening movement. And the amount of abduction required is perhaps even less when the voiceless segment is superimposed on a relatively unconstricted vocal tract as in intervocalic /h/ (cf. Hutters, 1984, for similar findings in Danish fricatives). The fact that in combinations of two voiceless segments a fairly large gesture occurs is also not surprising since the temporal constraints on the abductory/ adductory cycle are slackened. This slackening of constraints is particularly to be seen in the adductory phase which has often been observed to be more variable in form than the abductory phase. The abductory phase has a particular aerodynamic task to fulfil, whereas the adductory phase does not. In the light of observations of this kind it is probably arbitrary at this level of analysis whether a particular type of voiceless segment is described as /h/ or as pre-aspiration. Turning now from glottal to velar activity (for S1 only), the issue here is whether Pétursson's observation can be replicated that both phonemic /h/ as well as pre-aspiration may show slight lowering of the velum. The recording of velar activity (bottom panels of Figures 2 and 3) failed to reveal any peculiarities in the pre-aspiration phase: No evidence for lowering in the pre-aspiration phase was found. True, the soft palate was often lower during the pre-aspiration phase than during the subsequent occlusion but was in fact usually being raised during this phase, i.e. moving from the slightly lowered position for the preceding vowel

---

the statistical test for comparing with /h/ after pooling the pre-aspirates and voiceless nasals, thus increasing n from 9 to 18. This gave a significant difference between the pooled medial consonants and initial /h/ at $p<0.05$.

towards the high position for the plosive - all much as one might expect (e.g. Bell-Berti, 1980). In other words there is no difference between 'seppi/sepi' etc. in velar activity. Examination of word-initial /h/ revealed quite clearly that /h/ does not have a characteristic velar position. When a nasal is upcoming, as in 'hendi' velar position is already quite low in the /h/ (compare the position for word-initial /d/ in 'dembi') while when no nasal is in sight, the position is high, showing at the most some coarticulatory influence of the surrounding vowel. Thus it is difficult to find support for the identity of /h/ and pre-aspiration in velar behaviour.

3.2.2 Pre-aspirates vs. voiceless nasals

We now turn to a direct comparison of glottal activity in the pre-aspirates and the voiceless nasals.
Means and standard errors for three kinematic parameters are given for S1 in Figure 4: 1. peak glottal opening amplitude; 2. peak abduction velocity; 3. peak adduction velocity (timing parameters are considered afterwards). Both our hypothesis and Pétursson's would lead one to expect the activity to be quite similar in the two (groups of) sounds. Inspection of the ensemble averages in Figures 2 and 3 suggest that this is indeed the case, as far as form and size of the glottal gesture is concerned. However a two-way analysis of variance on 'hetta,seppi,henti,dempi' (i.e. the two leftmost pairs in each panel of Figure 4) shows that PGO, maximum abduction velocity and maximum adduction velocity are all significantly higher in the pre-aspirates than in the nasals ($p<0.01$).[7] Amplitude and velocity information of the transillumination technique should be treated with caution, however. This is underlined by the values for the third pair 'hitti, sempinn' in Figure 4. They were excluded from the analysis of variance as being less directly comparable than the other two pairs, but it is still noticeable that their values are virtually indistinguishable.[8] Moreover, for both of the supplementary subjects PGO

7 Note that 'hetta', the item with the largest opening amplitude, is not shown in the ensemble averages of Figures 2 and 3.

8 Caution is probably particularly in order for the third of the kinematic parameters shown in Figure 4 (maximum adduction velocity): There is some evidence in the ensemble averages of Figures 2 and 3 for velum-induced artefacts in the PGG curves (velar raising occurs roughly during glottal adduction, whereas velar lowering takes

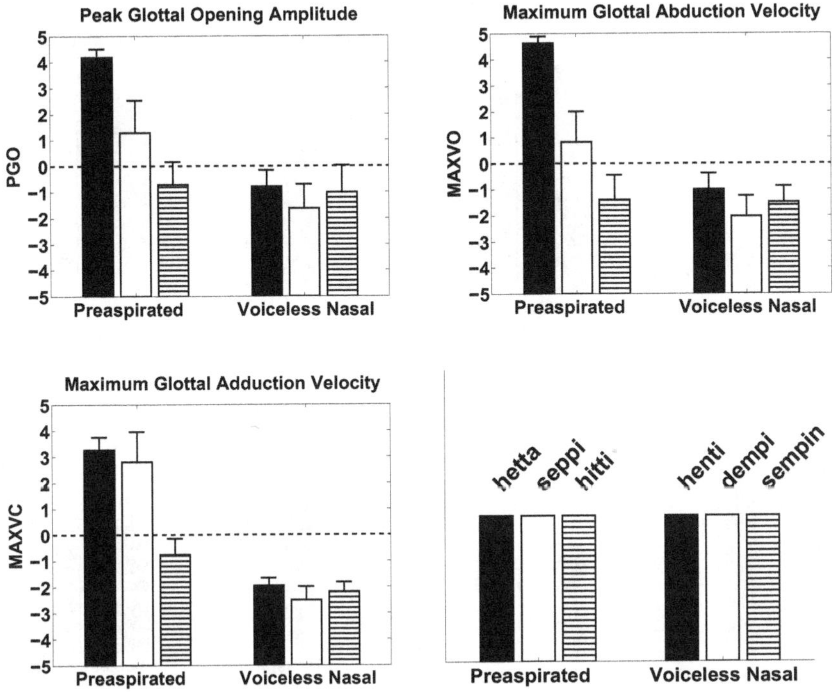

Figure 4. Means of glottal amplitude and velocity parameters for words with pre-aspirated plosives and voiceless nasals. Data normalized to zero mean and unit standard deviation in each block of repetitions. Bottom right panel indicates identity of each word in the three main panels. Error bars indicate standard error of mean (n=6).

amplitudes are marginally higher for the voiceless nasal 'henti' rather than the pre-aspirate 'hitti'. But these differences are nowhere near being significant in the signed rank test over 9 matched pairs (p-values of approx. 0.8 for both subjects).[9] And similarly for both the velocity parameters neither of these subjects showed any evidence at all of significant differences. The relationships in the *timing* of glottal activity can be approached with more confidence, however. Average results for the timing parameters are shown for S1 in Figure 5. There is one clear dif-

place sometime before glottal abduction).

9 As can be seen from Table 2 the mean amplitude differences do not exceed 0.2V for either subject. To put this in perspective, the standard deviation of the pairwise differences amounted to 0.8 (S2) and 0.9 (S3).

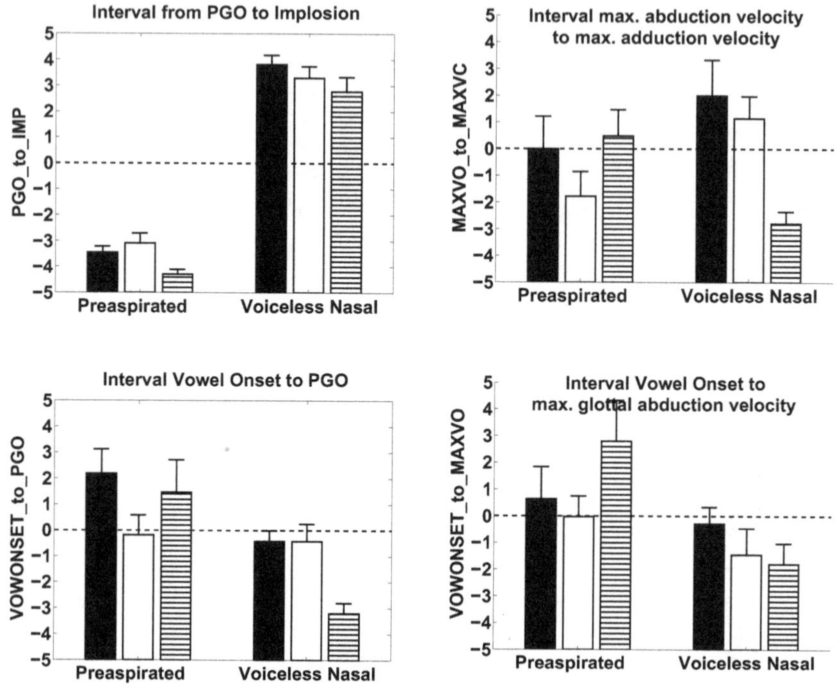

Figure 5. Means of glottal timing parameters for words with pre-aspirated plosives and voiceless nasals (normalized data). Other details as Figure 4 (i.e. from left to right bars are 'hetta, seppi, hitti, henti, dempi, sempinn')

ference, but also some interesting similarities between pre-aspirates and nasals.

Firstly, there is similarity with respect to the most basic durational parameter, namely the overall duration of the gesture. This was estimated by the interval from instant of maximum abduction velocity to instant of maximum adduction velocity (Figure 5, top right panel, for S1). This measure of the gesture duration was preferred to one based on onset and offset of the abduction movement because it appeared more stable with respect to fluctuation in the baseline of the transillumination signal. For none of the subjects did this measure show a significant difference between pre-aspirates and voiceless nasals.

The most striking difference on the other hand involves the interval from PGO to formation of the occlusion for the plosive. The top left panel of

Figure 5 gives a complete breakdown of all word-types for S1. Table 3 summarizes the results for all three subjects. While PGO more or less

Table 3. Means (in bold face) and sds of interval from Peak Glottal Opening to Implosion in ms. For S1 averaged over all three word-types per category (n=18). For S2 and S3 data only for 'hitti' and 'henti' (n=9).

	Duration		
Subject	S1	S2	S3
pre-aspirated	**10** ± 8.6	**-3** ± 4.5	**8** ± 13.6
voiceless nasal	**85** ± 13.5	**47** ± 9.2	**58** ± 22.7

coincides with the start of the oral occlusion phase in the pre-aspirates it is timed much earlier relative to this point in the voiceless nasal. The difference amounts to 50ms for S2 and S3, and 75ms for S1.

This is a natural consequence of the similarity in the overall duration of the glottal gesture in conjunction with the different structuring of the cluster outlined at the start of the results section, i.e. shorter occlusion duration for the voiceless nasal than for the pre-aspirate word-forms, and, conversely, longer duration of the voiceless nasal phase itself compared to the pre-aspiration phase. However, it does mean that our hypothesis cannot simply claim that a voiceless nasal results from placing a nasal in front of a pre-aspirate which remains otherwise unchanged (see discussion).

We were also particularly interested in determining whether our finding for German (referred to briefly at the end of section 2.1 above) that the interval from vowel onset to glottal abduction remained the same for an /st/ cluster and a single /t/ could be replicated in another language with different material (cf. Hoole et al., 1984). In this case it unfortunately proved impossible to reliably measure the point at which glottal abduction started due to the fluctuations in the baseline of the transillumination signal mentioned above. Nonetheless, for S1 the interval from vowel onset to the moment of maximal abduction velocity, and the interval from vowel onset to PGO were not significantly different in the two classes of sounds (see Figure 5, bottom panels), again excluding the rightmost pair for the reasons given above. For S3, too, no significant differences were found for either of these durational measures. S2, by contrast, did show significant differences (at $p<0.05$ for both parameters). Nevertheless, the differences between pre-aspirates and voiceless nasals amounted to less than 10ms for both parameters (which contrasts markedly with the just-mentioned 50ms difference in the timing of PGO relative to the start of the oral occlusion). Thus, it still seems possible to state, as for the earlier German results, that differently structured oral articulations are superimposed on rather similar glottal activity when viewed from the onset of the preceding vowel.

3.2.3 Voiced vs. voiceless nasals

The next group of results to be presented concerns velar and oral activity in the voiced and voiceless nasals. Under the hypothesis that the voiceless nasals are not themselves voiceless one might expect the nasals to be similar in velar activity and segmental duration. As already indicated in the discussion of the acoustic segment durations this was not borne out in the results. The voiceless nasals as measured from the audio signal (refer back to Table 1 and Figure 1) were clearly longer than the voiced ones ($p<0.01$ for all subjects). This agrees with the earlier acoustic measurements of Pétursson. An important further component in Pétursson's argument for the phonemicity of the voiceless nasals is that any opposition in the plosives following voiceless vs. voiced nasals is neutralized. The occlusion phases of the plosives are clearly voiceless in both cases, so the main interest attaches to the duration of the occlusion. Pétursson (1975) and, more recently, Jessen and Pétursson (1998) concluded that there was no consistent difference in the occlusion durations. This is not completely borne out by the present results. For S1 there is indeed no significant difference in the durations, but both S2 and S3 showed significantly shorter occlusion durations following the voiceless nasals ($p<0.01$ and $p<0.05$, respectively), i.e. a reciprocal adjustment almost compensating for the longer duration of the voiceless nasal segment itself (see Table 1 for details). Clearly the limited data for S2 and S3 do not provide strong grounds for rejecting the contention that the occlusion durations do not differ, but it might be interesting to follow up this issue with a much larger scale acoustic investigation of young speakers. Moreover, we will argue in the discussion section that even if the occlusion durations do not differ, this still does not necessarily need to imply the plosive opposition as a whole is completely neutralized. We now turn to the kinematic parameters of the velar gesture. These are

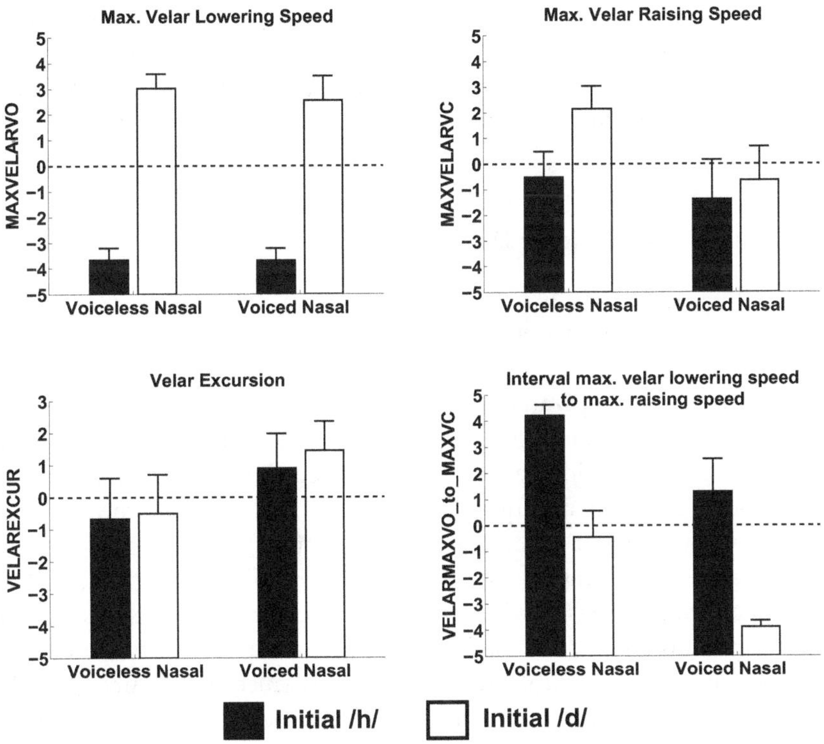

Figure 6. Means of kinematic parameters of velar activity for words with voiced and voiceless nasals (normalized data). In each panel from left to right the black bars (initial /h/) correspond to 'henti, hendi', the white bars (initial /d/) to 'dempi, dembi'. Other details as Figure 4

shown in Figure 6. There were no significant differences in maximum raising or lowering speed or in overall excursion based on a two-way analysis of variance of 'henti, dempi, hendi, dembi'. Taking the length of the interval between the positions of maximum lowering and raising speed as a measure of the length of the velar gesture there was also no significant difference in the analysis of variance performed on the raw data - slightly unexpectedly in view of the result obtained from the audio signal. Based on the normalized data, however, the difference was significant ($p<0.01$). This slightly equivocal result was probably due to the considerable anticipatory coarticulation in 'hendi/henti' which resulted in a slow lowering speed and rather inaccurate determination of the position of maximum lowering velocity (thus the patterns in the top left and bottom right panels are dominated by the difference between /h/-initial (black bars) and /d/-initial (white bars) words). A straight t-test on the raw data of 'dempi'/'dembi' turned out to be significant ($p<0.05$).

3.2.4 Plosive occlusions: Duration and air-pressure

In this final section of the results we consider two remaining characteristics of the plosive occlusions that have not been dealt with above.

Durations of pre-aspirated vs. unaspirated plosives: As mentioned in the introduction the duration of the occlusion phase of pre-aspirated and non-aspirated plosives has been of some interest with respect to the syllable-structure and quantity system of Icelandic. Accordingly, although not of central concern to our analysis of the pre-aspirates and voiceless nasal, we summarize the results here for the sake of completeness. Pooling the length of the occlusion from all three recordings for S1 for the pairs 'hitti/hiti' and 'seppi/sepi' no evidence for longer occlusions in the pre-aspirates could be found since both pairs differ by about 10ms, but in different directions (refer back to Table 1). For the supplementary speakers only the 'hitti/hiti' pair is available. For S2 the difference is clearly negligible. For S3 the pre-aspirate is actually about 16ms shorter (significant at $p<0.01$). Thus the results are in agreement with the other investigations quoted in the introduction since despite the traditional association of the pre-aspirates with long consonants there is no evidence that they actually have longer occlusions.

Intraoral air-pressure: From the air-pressure recording we measured the peak air pressure in the occlusion (see Figure 7). Dividing the words into four matched pairs differing in the presence vs. absence of a strong glottal abduction gesture a 2 x 4 analysis of variance on 'hitti, henti, seppi, dempi' vs. 'hiti, hendi, sepi, dembi' showed that the latter, i.e.

those without a large magnitude of glottal abduction have significantly higher peak air-pressures ($p<0.01$). Note that it is thus the plosives that would traditionally be regarded as fortis that have the lower pressures. The most plausible explanation for this result is that the expenditure of air before the oral occlusion in the pre-aspiration or voiceless nasal phases causes a temporary drop in sub-glottal pressure. Note that the effect may be somewhat stronger (i.e. lowest air-pressure of all) in the voiceless nasals because these have a longer period than the pre-aspirates in which glottal opening is combined with an unoccluded vocal tract.

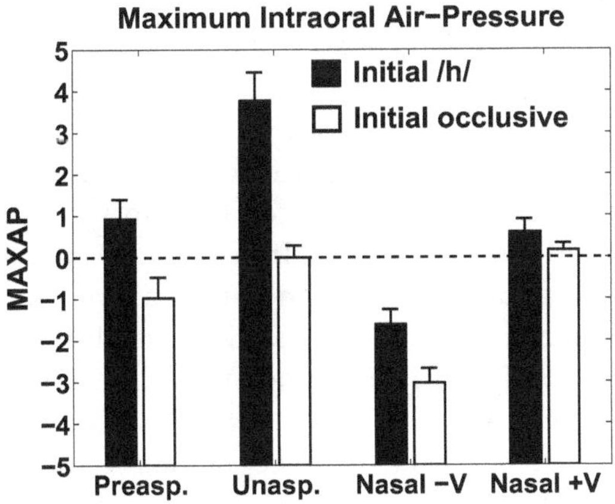

Figure 7. Means of maximum intraoral air-pressure in the occlusion phase (normalized data). From left to right, black bars (initial /h/) are 'hitti, hiti, henti, hendi', white bars (initial occlusive) are 'seppi, sepi, dempi, dembi'. Other details as Figure 4

4 Discussion of the results

The main points in the results can be summarized as follows:

- Pre-aspirated plosives and voiceless nasals have a very similar glottal gesture in terms of overall duration, and in the timing of its onset relative to the preceding vowel.
- No clear differences in magnitude of glottal abduction were found between these categories; they both tended to be larger than e.g.

prevocalic /h/ and unaspirated plosives.

- Duration of plosive occlusions was longer in the pre-aspirates than in the plosive following nasals.
- Duration of pre-aspiration was shorter than the duration of the voiceless nasal.
- Pre-aspirates and voiceless nasals differed radically in the timing of PGO relative to the start of the plosive occlusion (PGO timed earlier for voiceless nasals)
- Voiceless nasals were somewhat longer than the voiced nasals (both in terms of oral occlusion and duration of the velar gesture)

We will now review the immediate implications of the results for the original questions and hypotheses. In the following section the perspective is widened to take more recent literature into account.

Pétursson's arguments for analysing pre-aspirates as /h/+P received little support. Arguments in favour of the nasal hypothesis (voiceless nasals are not phonemic, but are a coarticulatory consequence of pre-aspiration) remain more equivocal. It might have simplified matters if the different nasals had proved identical in every respect except coarticulatory voicelessness. However the fact that they differ clearly in length, for example, obviously does not prevent them from being allophones of the same phoneme.

The fact that glottal behaviour was very similar in the pre-aspirate and voiceless nasal cases does not necessarily mean that both cases must have the same number of phonemic segments, i.e. two in Pétursson's view. This is particularly the case if the voiceless nasal is accepted as underlying voiced, with [ʰp] and [m̥p] thus qualitatively similar to cases such as [pʰ] and [pl̥] in English and other languages (see below for further discussion of this possible analogy; see e.g. Ridouane et al. (2007) for recent discussion of an extensive range of cases illustrating the relationship between the number of segments and the number of observable glottal abduction gestures).

The probably more crucial issue involves the changing relationships between glottal and oral activity: When the plosive is preceded by a nasal it becomes shorter. This is in itself a trivial observation, yet the effect is the same on both pre-aspirated and unaspirated plosives (see Table 1). Should one then expect the glottal gesture in the pre-aspirates to undergo similar modification, i.e. should in particular the position of PGO relative to acoustic onset of the plosive remain (relatively) the same? Not necessarily, if one accepts the point of view we developed on the basis of the German material (Hoole et al., 1984), namely that the speech mechanism reorganizes oral articulations more readily than glottal ones. Moreover, analysis of the laryngeal gesture associated with onset clusters (Hoole, 2006b) suggests that the gesture is organized to reflect the aerodynamic demands of the onset as a whole. A somewhat similar account may be appropriate here. The fact that oral activity was rearranged while glottal activity was not, could, at some level, represent an economy of effort; linguistically, the job of the motor system is to maintain the distinction between e.g. 'dempi' and 'dembi'. This can be accomplished more reliably by devoicing the nasal completely, and at the same time perhaps more economically by using the glottal activity pattern for normal pre-aspirates. In a sense, it may simply not be appropriate to ask which segment the devoicing gesture 'belongs' to (see Lodge, 2007, for a non-segmental perspective on aspiration in Icelandic).

Our proposed account does, however, leave open at least one perspective that would warrant further exploration: In the present experiments the pre-aspirates and voiceless nasals never showed more than one glottal opening peak. However, it cannot be completely ruled out that either or both of these sound categories underlyingly consist of two strongly overlapped glottal gestures (Munhall and Löfqvist, 1992), that may only become visible individually at very slow speech rates. Here we are arguing for a basic similarity in the glottal gesture for pre-aspirates and voiceless nasals, so it would constitute evidence against this hypothesis if it turned out that these sound categories behave differently over variation in speech rate with respect to the glottal movement patterns.

A last argument in favour of the plausibility of our view of the voiceless nasals is that the same phenomenon, i.e. one of coarticulation, in a different context has traditionally led to an analysis equivalent to the one we are proposing. In English, in such pairs as 'plead/bleed', one could also assert that the phonological contrast is carried by the voicing of the liquid. Yet few voices have been raised in favour of voiceless /l/ as a phoneme of English.

Here one could also venture the hypothesis that in English 'pea' vs. 'plea' a constant glottal articulation is combined with reorganized oral articulation, so that for example peak glottal opening occurs at a different time relative to the release of the /p/ occlusion in the two words.[10] If our approach is accepted a considerable simplification of the Icelandic sound system results. To be completely coherent however the analysis would have to be extended to the voiceless liquids, which are distributed similarly to the voiceless nasals. The Icelandic sound-system also becomes more typically European (cf. again Werner's (1963) reservations when proposing a rather "unEuropean" system for Faroese) since, in addition to the absence of voiceless continuants, we now have two series of stops with a fairly free distribution if we accept an allophonic rule for place of aspiration. Previously, the aspirated stops were restricted to word-initial position, being here post-aspirated.[11]

To conclude this discussion of the results, we would like to consider briefly the patterns of anticipatory velar coarticulation observable in our data.

Assuming that the production of the voiceless nasal segments requires coordination of velar, laryngeal and oral activity it might be natural to expect these three systems to be constrained to act as a unit. Since we were unable to record velar and laryngeal activity simultaneously in this experiment we cannot attack this question as directly as we would wish. However it is quite apparent from our recordings that the factor most strongly influencing velar activity is the presence or absence of an /h/ at the beginning of the word containing the nasal. Bell-Berti (1980) has pointed out that some attempts to demonstrate a feature-spreading model of anticipatory velar coarticulation have failed to take into account the different intrinsic velar heights of purely oral sounds, particularly vowels. There is a great deal of merit in this observation. However, even when this is taken into account, the amount of velar depression by the time the /h/ is reached appears so large that it is tempting to think that its specification for velar position is so weak that some feature-spreading is occurring. This experiment was not designed to investigate the viability of feature-spreading as such. For the moment we would

10 This issue has now been looked at in detail for German material in Hoole, 2006b. The patterns of reorganization were actually somewhat more complex than the one originally assumed here. But it was possible to unify them under the assumption that the speaker actively plans to generate a longer period of voicelessness following release of /p/ in /pl/, than following the release of singleton /p/.

11 Note that Northern Icelandic also has post-aspirated stops where the present corpus has unaspirated ones, e.g. in 'hiti'.

simply join Al Bamerni (1984) in suspecting that compared to other articulatory systems velar activity is subject to fewer (or different) constraints.

5 General discussion

The discussion throughout the introduction and the presentation of the results has centered very much on the ideas presented in Pétursson's many papers, this being the only body of work giving a comprehensive experimental perspective on the relevant phenomena.
However, in more recent years, for the majority of those who have worked on Icelandic sound structure our basic contention is probably neither particularly radical nor controversial, namely that the voicelessness of the nasals in the contexts examined here does not motivate the assumption of nasal phonemes in Icelandic.
Thus, in a more recent paper arguing for voiceless nasal phonemes in Icelandic, Jessen and Pétursson (1998) clearly regard themselves as swimming against the current when they state (p. 43) that *"despite the mainstream opinion it is possible and in several ways desirable to ascribe distinctive status to the voiceless nasals of Icelandic"*, and that the majority view favours a derivational account of nasal devoicing that is closely related to analysis of pre-aspiration. Where our account still differs from the so-called mainstream phonological approach is in the role assigned to coarticulatory processes. We contend that this still has the potential to short-circuit much of the discussion since in this perspective nasal devoicing simply does not need accounting for in the phonology, once one has a laryngeal-oral coordination relation for pre-aspirated plosives as a point of departure. This is essentially identical to Browman and Goldstein's (1986) motivation for a gestural account of laryngeal contrasts. Thus, just by way of example, in a recent analysis within the framework of Optimality Theory Ringen (1999) needs to arrive at a representation that associates [spread glottis] with both the plosive and the preceding sonorant. The wider point is that this may be unnecessary if phonological representations incorporate a concept of time that goes beyond what Gafos (2002) has recently referred to as the 'trivial' concept of time, i.e. one restricted to serial order (see also Gafos et al., 2010), though admit-

tedly we are not going to resolve such an issue here with limited data on just a few speakers of Icelandic.

To round off this review of the more recent discussion, it is important to come back to the above-mentioned paper of Jessen and Pétursson (1998), since they raise a number of cogent points that deserve detailed consideration.

First of all, they point out that discussion of the existence of voiceless nasals (and other sonorants) has tended to neglect their occurrence in syllable-initial position[12]. This is certainly an objection that can be applied to our own work here. These sounds are undoubtedly phonetically interesting. Although often referred to as voiceless, it appears from a recent study (based on further material from the recordings of S2 and S3 used here) that they often involve only a rather small amount of glottal abduction and may actually show uninterrupted - but non-modal - voicing (Bombien, 2006, see there for further references). This is a rather different situation from the voiceless sonorants before plosives, which appear to be really completely voiceless, and where the amplitude of glottal opening (extending of course into the following plosive) is clearly extensive. We will leave as an open question here whether they should be given phonemic status or analyzed as /h/+sonorant. The latter analysis has a tradition extending back to Haugen, but, as Jessen and Pétursson note, such sequences would, if adopted, sit rather awkwardly in the rest of the Icelandic sound system. It might prove interesting to follow these sounds over the next few decades, because the non-modal voicing could be a hint of a change in progress in their realization.

The other major point raised by Jessen and Pétursson concerns the appositeness of regarding voiceless sonorants before plosives as a parallel phenomenon to devoicing of sonorants after voiceless sounds in languages such as English, German and in fact Icelandic itself (Hoole, 1987, 1999a, 2006b).

The first argument they use in this connection is that sonorant devoicing is a gradient phenomenon in English etc. since the the amount of devoicing varies with the preceding sound, e.g. plosive, fricative, fricative-plosive cluster, whereas the sounds are categorically and completely voiceless in Icelandic. However, the strength of this argument is diffi-

12 A contrastive example: 'nýta' [ni:ta] (to use) 'hnýta' [n̥i:ta] (to knot), from Bombien (2006)

cult to judge, since there is probably simply not a comparable range of contexts in Icelandic that could allow gradient behaviour to be revealed. A rather interesting further observation made by them is that native speakers of Icelandic are not aware of devoicing of sonorants in cases like /pl/ any more than phonetically naive English speakers are, but that they are aware of something like voicelessness in the reverse case - which hence should perhaps be regarded as having a different status. Finally, they raise a point that we would prefer to see from a completely different perspective, but where, paradoxically, we are actually very much in sympathy with the underlying motivation for the direction they are trying to take. In their view, the plosive opposition in pairs like 'henti/hendi' is completely neutralized, i.e. both are voiceless unaspirated, and show an occlusion duration that is very similar (though note that the latter assumption is qualified somewhat by our findings for S2 and S3; cf. section 3.2.3 above), whereas this complete neutralization is probably not present in the more familiar cases such as /pl/ vs. /bl/ etc. Their point of view must assign the glottal gesture exclusively to the nasal (or other sonorant), whereas we are taking the perspective that the basic coordination relation at issue here is the one for a pre-aspirated plosive - even if it does become modified for the cluster compared to the pre-aspirated case. In our view, then, the plosives are, of course, radically different. This is where resolution is difficult: "You pays your money and takes your choice". Why did we nonetheless just indicate that we were in sympathy with the more general motivation of their argument? Part of their motivation for favouring the phonemicity of the voiceless nasals is that it avoids the necessity for, in their view, an unduly abstract phonological representation, i.e. one involving "*the assumption that the voicelessness of sonorants is derived by characteristics of the following stop that are accessible not in concrete phonetic, but only abstract phonological terms*" (Jessen and Pétursson, 1998, p. 43).

This is in fact precisely the motivation for the coarticulatory perspective put forward here: we assume that we do indeed have a very concrete difference between the stops, and obtain the voiceless nasals by getting as much mileage as possible from the application of very general and unabstract principles of coordinated behaviour. Nobody would deny that the temporal dimension is crucial to speech. In fact, all human behaviour is probably built up on principles of temporal coordination. The widely diverging views for the small problem discussed here may simply reflect the fact that principles of temporal coordination have not yet been well integrated into phonological representations, and, more surprisingly, often not even into phonetic accounts.

References

Al Bamerni, A. (1984). Speech rate and velar control. In Cohen, A. and van den Broecke, M. P. R., editors, *Abstracts of the 10th International Congress of Phonetic Sciences*, page 464.

Bell-Berti, F. (1980). Velopharyngeal function: A spatio-temporal model. *Haskins SR*, 63/4:41 ff.

Bombien, L. (2006). Voicing alterations in Icelandic - a photoglottographic and acoustic investigation. *AIPUK*, 37:63–82.

Browman, C. and Goldstein, L. (1986). Towards an articulatory phonology. *Phonology Yearbook*, 3:219–252.

Gafos, A. (2002). A grammar of gestural coordination. *Natural Language and Lingustic Theory*, 20(1):169–337.

Gafos, A., Hoole, P., Roon, K., and Zeroual, C. (2010). Variation in timing and phonological grammar in Moroccan Arabic clusters. In Fougeron, C., Kühnert, B., d'Imperio, M., and Vallé, N., editors, *Laboratory Phonology 10: Variation, Detail and Representation*. Mouton de Gruyter, Berlin/New York.

Garnes, S. (1973). Phonetic evidence supporting a phonological analysis. *Journal of Phonetics*, 1:273–283.

Haugen, E. (1958). The phonemics of modern Icelandic. *Language*, 34:55–88.

Hoole, P. (1987). Velar and glottal activity in a speaker of Icelandic. In *Proceedings of the 11th International Congress of Phonetic Sciences*, volume 3, pages 31–34, Tallinn, Estonia. Academy of Sciences of the ESSR.

Hoole, P. (1999a). Laryngeal Coarticulation. Section A: Coarticulatory investigations of the devoicing gesture. In Hardcastle, W. J. and Hewlett, N., editors, *Coarticulation: Theory, Data and Techniques*, pages 105–121. Cambridge University Press, Cambridge.

Hoole, P. (1999b). Techniques for investigating laryngeal articulation and the voice-source. Section A: Investigation of the devoicing gesture. In Hardcastle, W. J. and Hewlett, N., editors, *Coarticulation: Theory, Data and Techniques*, pages 294–300. Cambridge University Press, Cambridge.

Hoole, P. (2006a). *Experimental studies of laryngeal articulation. Appendix: Velar and glottal activity in Icelandic.* Unpublished habilitation thesis, Ludwig-Maximilians-Universität, Munich. http://www.phonetik.uni-muenchen.de/~hoole/pdf/habilicelandic.pdf [accessed May 1, 2010].

Hoole, P. (2006b). *Experimental studies of laryngeal articulation. Part 2: Larygeal-Oral coordination in consonant sequences.* Unpublished habilitation thesis, Ludwig-Maximilians-Universität, Munich. http://www.phonetik.uni-muenchen.de/~hoole/pdf/habilpgg_chap_all.pdf [accessed May 1, 2010].

Hoole, P., Pompino-Marschall, B., and Dames, M. (1984). Glottal timing in German voiceless occlusives. In Van der Broecke, M. and Cohen, A., editors, *Prooceedings of the 10th International Congress of Phonetic Sciences,* pages 309–403, Utrecht, The Netherlands.

Hutters, B. (1976). Problems in the use of the photoelectric glottograph. *Annual Report of the Institute of Phonetics of the University of Copenhagen,* 10:274–312.

Hutters, B. (1984). Vocal fold adjustments in Danish voiceless obstruent production. *Annual Reports of the Institute of Phonetics, University of Copenhagen,* 18:293–385.

Jessen, M. and Pétursson, M. (1998). Voiceless nasal phonemes in Icelandic. *Journal of the International Phonetic Association,* 28:43–53.

Künzel, H. (1979). Röntgenvideographische Evaluierung eines Photoelektrischen Verfahrens zur Messung der Velumhöhe beim Sprechen. *Folia Phoneatrica,* 31:153–166.

Lodge, K. (2007). Timing, segmental status and aspiration in Icelandic. *Transactions of the Philological Society,* 105(1):66–104.

Löfqvist, A. and Yoshioka, H. (1980). Laryngeal activity in Icelandic obstruent production. *Haskins SR,* 63:275–292.

Löfqvist, A. and Yoshioka, H. (1980). Laryngeal activity in Swedish obstruent clusters. *Journal of the Acoustical Society of America,* 63:792–801.

Munhall, K. and Löfqvist, A. (1992). Gestural aggregation in speech: laryngeal gestures. *Journal of Phonetics,* 20:111–126.

Pétursson, M. (1972). La préaspiration en islandaise moderne. Examen de sa réalisation phonétique chez deux sujets. *Studia Linguistica,* 26:61–80.

Pétursson, M. (1973a). L'origine des phonèmes nasals et liquides sourds et du [h] postvocalique de l'islandaise moderne. *Orbis,* 22:335–342.

Pétursson, M. (1973b). Phonologie des consonnes nasales en islandais moderne. *La Linguistique,* 9:115–138.

Pétursson, M. (1975). Examen expérimental de la réalistion phonétique des nasales sourdes de l'islandaise moderne. In Dahlstedt, K.-H., editor, *The Nordic Languages and Modern Linguistics*, volume 2, pages 634–653. Almqvist & Wiksell, Stockholm.

Pétursson, M. (1976). Aspiration et activité glottale. Examen expérimental à partir de consones islandaises. *Phonetica*, 33:169–198.

Ridouane, R., Hoole, P., and Fuchs, S. (2007). Laryngeal behavior in voiceless words and sentences: a photoelectroglottographic study. In Trouvain, J. and Barry, W., editors, *Proceedings of the 16th International Congress of Phonetic Sciences [ICPhS XVI]*, pages 2049–2052, August.

Ringen, C. O. (1999). Aspiration, preaspiration, deaspiration, sonorant devoicing and spirantization in Icelandic. *Nordic Journal of Linguistics*, 22:137–156.

Werner, O. (1963). Aspiration und stimmlose Nasale/Liquide im phonologischen System des Färingischen. *Phonetica*, 9:79–107.

Articulation Beyond the Usual: Evaluating the Fastest German Speaker under Laboratory Conditions

STEFANIE JANNEDY
SUSANNE FUCHS
MELANIE WEIRICH

Abstract: It is assumed that the rate at which speakers articulate is constrained by physiological factors such as the mass of an articulator and the distance an articulator must travel, by linguistic factors such as the utterance's phonetic complexity and by cognitive factors. We carried out an articulatory study using Electromagnetic Articulography (EMA) with a simultaneous acoustic recording of a single speaker who has practiced various tongue twisters for more than 40 years. Acoustic results indicate that our speaker can achieve up to 10 syllables per second in some tongue twisters. Comparing the articulatory results in normal versus fast speech it turned out that our subject either reduces movement amplitudes or uses a combination of reduction in movement amplitude and peak velocity, depending on the articulator involved and the particular sound. Although in fast speech movement amplitudes are generally reduced, they are still relatively large. Thus, we conclude that maintaining large movement amplitudes may be one strategy to avoid speech errors or articulatory reorganization, both of which are common in fast speech.[1]

1 Introduction

In this work we report on our investigation of the highly practiced, super fast speech of Dr. Georg Winter, who is the undisputed fastest speaker

1 A training tongue twister for you Bernd - to become the next ultrafast speaker: Bester Bobby pustet blaue Blubberblasen und plappert blumige Balladen mit beiden Beinen im Badesee baumelnd.

of German tongue twisters and who has won several speaking competitions on German TV. We conducted an Electromagnetic Articulography (EMA) study with the aim of better understanding the underlying mechanisms of competing requirements: speaking extremely fast without losing the linguistically relevant acoustic information necessary to recover the message. The aim of this paper is not to describe changes in the acoustics due to faster rates of speech in general, but to explore the articulatory mechanisms by which different types of sounds are realized under very fast rate conditions.

Speaking requires an enormously complex interplay between cognitive and physiological factors: meaning has to be transformed into articulatory movements. Just how exactly this interplay between cognition and the transformation into coordinated articulatory movements occurs remains speculative. We can, however, measure how fast a well-trained speaker can recite tongue twisters of differing phonetic complexity. We believe that in highly practiced speech, such as the recitation of poems, prayers or tongue twisters, much of the linguistic planning is removed, so that a speaker can focus entirely on the mastery and coordination of the articulatory movements. In this paper, we investigate the acoustic duration of syllables and the kinematic patterns of the human articulatory apparatus at extremely fast rates of speech and compare them to a control condition in which the speaker spoke at a self-defined normal rate.

In phonology, consonants are defined in terms of their place and manner of articulation, and their voicing status. (Note that voicing is not considered as a factor in this paper.) Here, we are looking at the physical, physiological and biomechanical foundations of speech sounds and therefore refer to the gestures and the articulators themselves rather than to their place of articulation. The articulators are the part of the vocal apparatus that move, that gain or lose velocity, and that are actively controlled in the production of speech sounds. As such, they contribute to the differences in speech rate. Manner characteristics of fricatives, stops etc. are studied in terms of the different control mechanisms of the articulatory gestures.

1.1 Biomechanical and weight properties

In comparison to most other parts of the body, speech articulators such as the tongue or the lips consist of soft tissue only and do not involve bony structure. This property makes these articulators extremely fast, since they are light in mass and very flexible. Moreover, normal speech is so fast already that online auditory feedback, which usually has a latency of at least 100 ms (Honda et al., 2002), is not possible for each individual unit of sound. The jaw, which consists of muscles and bony structure, is the heaviest in weight, and is therefore the slowest articulator. Its critical contribution to the production of sounds is still a matter of debate. For instance, Articulatory Phonology (Browman and Goldstein, 1990, 1992) supposes that the jaw is not an independent articulator but a component articulator for all tongue gestures and lip aperture and serves as a general regulator for rhythmic patterns. A greater jaw opening leads to greater amplitude of the signal and also to more extreme formant values in vowels (Beckman et al., 1995; Beckman and Edwards, 1994). Mooshammer et al. (2007), however, argue that in addition to the tongue tip, the jaw position is crucial in sibilants like /s/ and in the production of /t/. Thus, as the tongue tip is released, the lower incisors serve as an obstacle to the air stream to enhance the intensity of the burst. Note that a high jaw position for /t/ is probably only relevant when a perceptually salient burst is required.

The main articulator, the tongue, consists of many interdigitated muscle fibers resulting in a complex biomechanical structure (Takemoto, 2001). Although the tongue moves as a whole within the vocal tract, some regions of the tongue may be partially decoupled (Lindblom, 1989), that is, they move somewhat more independently than other parts, e.g. in very rapid tongue tip movements as they occur in flap productions. The complex nature of this biomechanical structure is often discussed with respect to the tongue dorsum/tongue back looping movement found in the productions of velar stops (Perrier et al., 2003). Loops in a sequence such as /aka/ involve not only a strong vertical, but also a horizontal movement component, although the latter is not required from a perceptual point of view.

Given the weight and biomechanical considerations we attribute to the articulators, we suppose that depending on the articulators involved in the production of speech sounds, some sounds can be rendered faster than others. Our predictions are:

1. Slowest: Tongue twisters involving the jaw in synchrony with the tongue tip, e.g. /t, s, ʃ /, have the slowest speech rate, since the jaw is the heaviest articulator.

2. Intermediate: Tongue twisters involving looping patterns as in /k/ have a relatively slow speech rate, because of the biomechanical properties involved in their production.

3. Fastest: Tongue twisters involving tongue tip or lip movements, e.g. /p, l/, have the fastest speech rate, since the tongue tip and the lips are light and thus relatively fast moving articulators.

Note though that allophonic variants such as a /ɾ/ as a possible realization of /t/ would fall under the third prediction rather than the first as we assume that the involvement of the jaw is minimal in comparison to a fully realized [t], which may have a prominent burst.

1.2 Different control strategies in selected phones

Besides the intrinsic duration distinctions of vowels (all things being equal, low vowels are intrinsically longer than high vowels), it is also frequently found that consonants or parts of consonants are intrinsically longer than others. For example, in general, voiceless velar stops have a longer Voice Onset Time (VOT) than bilabial stops. These differences can be attributed to a variety of articulatory and aerodynamic factors (see Cho and Ladefoged, 1999, for an overview).

One can also stipulate that the longer the sound, the more complex or more difficult it is to realize. But what exactly does more complex or more difficult mean? We will concentrate on two examples: 1. the production of voiceless stops versus fricatives, and 2. the production of phonologically complex consonant clusters and affricates versus singletons.

From a motor control point of view it has been hypothesized on the basis of kinematic data that the articulatory gestures involved in the production of stops are planned towards a target beyond the contact location

(Löfqvist and Gracco, 1997; Fuchs et al., 2006). Thus, stops are not controlled via a fine positioning of the tongue at the palate (or the lower lip at the upper lip in the case of bilabials). They are controlled by means of a reference, which automatically blocks the tongue's movement at the required location and leads to the intended salient acoustic closure. Moreover, the impact of the tongue at the palate may lead to shortening of the whole gesture. Such an effect has been modeled by means of a biomechanical tongue model in Fuchs and Perrier (2005). In terms of stability and simplicity, such a control strategy seems more efficient in comparison to the control necessary for a fine-tuned positioning of the tongue at the palate as is required for alveolar fricatives (Fuchs et al., 2006).

Fricatives require more finely tuned motor control as a constriction needs to be formed while the air pressure is high enough to establish turbulence downstream of the constriction. Alveolar fricatives are acquired later in children's speech development in comparison to sounds that do not require such fine-tuned motor control (Locke and Pearson, 1992). Patients who suffer from sensori-motor coordination impairments seem to have the most problems with the finely controlled articulation of /s/ and /ʃ/ (for a review, see Fuchs et al., 2007). On the basis of kinematic results, Fuchs et al. (2006) conclude that fricatives are planned with an articulatory target at the lateral margins of the palate in order to create a narrow midsagittal grove as a prerequisite for the production of turbulent noise, the most prominent acoustic characteristic of fricatives. In order to achieve this, a rather precise tongue and jaw position is required. In addition, fricatives are generally longer in duration than stops, although the movement amplitude is larger in stops than in fricatives. Given the precision necessary for the production of fricatives we extend the first hypothesis to take into account the fine motor control needed in the production of such sounds:

4. Tongue twisters involving voiceless stops are realized at a faster speech rate than those involving voiceless fricatives.

An added layer of complexity and difficulty is encountered in the comparison of phonological structures containing simple onsets or codas with structures that have complex onsets or codas. Further, affricates are articulatorily just as complex as consonant sequences even though phonologically they are often considered as a single segment (Fuchs and Koenig, 2009). We hypothesize that:

5. Tongue twisters involving a complex syllable structure are realized with a slower speech rate in comparison to those with a simpler phonological structure.

We will evaluate our fast speech data with regard to the hypotheses presented above.

1.3 Speech rates

A normal speech rate is defined as the speed at which our speaker was leisurely producing the text without trying to be extra fast or extra slow or overly deliberate. Normal rates, however, can also display articulatory reductions that lead to changes in the supposed canonical string and result in a phonetic output that includes consonant cluster reductions or fewer syllables. Kohler (1989) speculates on possible derivations (through deletions, assimilations and other reductive processes), starting with a canonical string, an idealized phonological form, and ending with a fairly reduced pronunciation typical for casual speech (e.g. *mit dem Wagen* 'with the car' [mɪt dem ˈvaːgən] can be realized as [mɪm ˈvaːŋ]). Casual speech can obviously be rendered at different speech rates depending on the communicative requirement. At faster rates, the speaker may be more or less accurate in the execution of motor patterns. In a taxonomy of speaking styles, casual contrasts with a more formal speaking style, and both of these speaking styles may be slower or faster. Nevertheless, some reduction phenomena that are supposedly caused by the rate of speech are also found in casual, less carefully produced speech.
It seems that a distinction is necessary between casual speech and fast speech (Lindblom, 1989) even though the literature on articulatory reduction often seems to make no distinction between these two. It is known that faster rates of speech can cause modifications to the standard timing relationships among speech gestures (Davidson, 2006; Munhall and Löfqvist, 1992), often leading to overlapping or even hiding of a gesture so that as a consequence, the resulting acoustic output does not contain audible traces of the originally intended articulatory configuration (Browman and Goldstein, 1990). In addition, it has been pointed

out that fast speech rates may not affect all phones to the same extent (Pfitzinger, 2001). Here we define fast speech as that rendered much faster than is common in normal conversation. Some research has focused on reduction phenomena of German fast speech (Kohler, 1989; Jannedy, 1995), whereby vowel reduction and other articulatory restructuring can alter the acoustic signals in significant ways. Ideally though, fast speech displays the same degree of articulatory precision as normal rates of speech.

1.4 Our speaker: Georg Winter

Georg Winter was born and raised in Hamburg, which is located in the northern part of Germany where some people still speak the highly endangered Low German dialect. Growing up in Hamburg, Georg Winter learned to speak Low German from the people around him, and to this date, his speech has several undeniable features of this dialect. When not paying attention, he produces /s/ before /t/ as in "Stein" *stone* or before /p/ as in "Sport" *sport* as [st] or [sp] rather than as [ʃt] or [ʃp] respectively, which is uncommon for more standard varieties of German. He also displays the spirantization of final /b d g/ that is typical for this dialect and realizes "Hamburg" as [hambʊaç]. In this dialect area the voiced or flapped version of /t/ is common.

As a child he suffered from a lisp and started practicing tongue twisters to overcome his speech problem. Georg Winter's assumption is that the muscles necessary for speaking (tongue, lips and any other muscle involved in articulation) can be trained just like any other muscle structure in the body.

Over the last five to six years, Georg Winter has made a name for himself as a speech-athlete, having had numerous appearances on game shows and talk shows, competing with other German 'speech' professionals such as rappers, talk show hosts or news anchors for the title of "Germany's fastest speaker". He is the undisputed master of his discipline, producing the most difficult tongue twisters with great precision and speed, which comes as no surprise, since he has been practicing his technique for over forty years now. At a normal rate, Georg Winter performed the texts rather expressively and with rhetorical skill. He paid much attention to grouping strings into felicitous prosodic units, pausing when necessary and using gaze and gesture to support the realization of the tongue twisters. Most of the material that he recites so rapidly was written by Georg Winter himself, and a small set of these tongue twisters is listed in the appendix. He trained himself to speak fast without losing information, that is, without altering the signal beyond recognition. An informal comprehension test revealed that in fact, Georg Winter's fastest tongue twisters are utterly incomprehensible to listeners who are hearing the tongue twisters for the first time and who have no further pragmatic cues as to what the speaker is saying. However, repeated exposure (listening to the stimuli repeatedly during labeling, zooming in on single words or phrases) and especially previous knowledge of the content of the tongue twister yielded a very high comprehension of his speech.

Georg Winter has held classes at schools, teaching students how to articulate tongue twisters extremely quickly. He describes the first step of his technique as learning articulatory templates, using simple syllables such as 'da', whereby he assigns such a 'da' to every syllable of a tongue twister and then adjusts the duration of these syllables in accordance with the stress requirements: if the syllable is lexically stressed, the syllable is sustained a little longer than when it is not stressed. He diligently practices the articulatory patterns, opening and closing the vocal tract by means of the template method. The next step in practicing ultra-fast speech is to introduce rhythmic alternations on these strings, even though the resulting rhythm may be linguistically infelicitous with regard to the message that is being realized. Only when these rhythmic alternations have been mastered are the actual sounds of the words practiced. It is possible that he acquired his rhythmic awareness through practicing and playing the piano as a child and doing finger exercises.

We chose to study Mr. Winter's speech by means of EMA to test whether his articulation reveals certain strategies especially suitable for rendering ultra-fast speech. To achieve fast rates of speech, several speaker-specific articulatory strategies have been reported. Among them are the reduction of movement amplitude, the increase in movement velocity and the amount of inter-gestural overlap (Byrd and Tan, 1996). We assume that Mr. Winter's speech reveals some peculiarities, since he realizes tongue twisters in an ultra-fast way without the normally expected speech errors.

2 Methodology

In this section, we will describe the recording procedure, the speech material, and the analysis methods that we have employed for the acoustic and articulatory data exploration.

2.1 Experimental design

We conducted an EMA experiment in which we asked Georg Winter to recite 6 tongue twisters (in random order) 5 times at a normal rate and then 5 times at the fastest possible rate (6 tongue twisters x 5 repetitions x 2 speech rates = 60 experimental trials total). The texts (which he also knew by heart) appeared on a screen located outside of the sound-proofed room where recording was performed and were visible through a window. Articulatory recordings were carried out using a 2D Electromagnetic Articulograph (Carstens Medizinelektronik, AG 100). Two sensors (one on the upper incisors and one on the bridge of the nose) served as references to compensate for head movements. Three more sensors were glued to the tongue: one at approximately 1 cm from the tongue tip, one on the tongue back and one between them on the tongue dorsum. Another sensor was placed below the lower incisors in order to track jaw movements, and two additional sensors were glued to the upper and the lower lips to record lip movements (see Figure 1).
The sampling frequency of the processed articulatory data was 200 Hz, and that of the acoustics 48 kHz. After the recordings, the sensor on the tongue tip was removed and the contour of the palate was recorded by moving this sensor along the palate from back to front. The articulatory data were pre-processed including correction algorithms for head movement, filtering of the data (low pass filter: bandwidth of 18 Hz with a damping of 50 dB at 52 Hz), and rotation and translation of the positional data to the occlusion plane. The occlusion plane was defined by means of two coils glued on a custom-made t-bar gripped by the subject between his teeth. In EMA, the y-axis refers to the vertical dimension and the occlusion plane defines the zero line at the y-axis. Velocities of the articulatory coils were additionally calculated as the derivatives of the sensor data. These signals were low pass filtered with a bandwidth of 15 Hz and a damping of 50 dB at 25 Hz. During the pre-processing

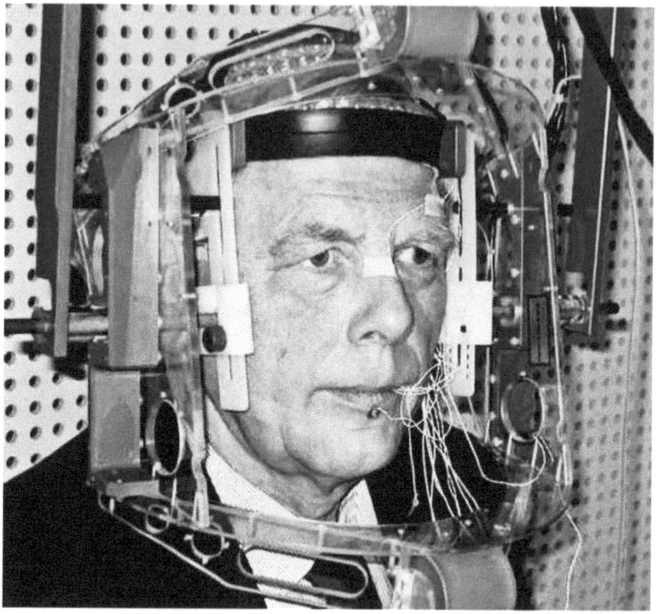

Figure 1. Georg Winter before the recording session.

procedure we made sure that the filter characteristics did not affect our results regarding the tangential velocity signals of the data.
In order to verify the quality of our data, we inspected the tilt values. Since the tongue dorsum sensor showed relatively high standard deviations, it will not be considered any further in the articulatory analysis.

2.2 Speech material

Our corpus contains 6 tongue twisters (see appendix, based on Winter, 2006). We selected them based on the consonants most frequently occurring in them. For ease of recognition, we gave them names based on the type of consonant that we are interested in studying. An overview of the different tongue twisters, the number of analyzed items per tongue twister at both rates, all target words and phonemes under investigation, their vowel context and the corresponding articulators is given in Table 1.

Table 1. Information about target sequences in relevant tongue twisters.

No.	Tongue twister	Number of samples	Target words	Sound sequence	V context	C articulator
1	tC-twister	normal: 50 fast: 50	Po**tsd**amer	/tsd/	/ɔ/, /a/	combination
			Postku**tsch**er	/tʃ/	/ʊ/, /ɐ/	
			Co**ttb**usser	/tb/	/ɔ/, /ʊ/	
			Postku**tsch-k**asten	/tʃk/	/ʊ/, /a/	
			pu**tzt**	/tst/	/ʊ/	
2	k-twister	normal: 45 fast: 45	Ka**k**ao Ka**k**adu Ka**k**alatsche	/k/	/a/, /a/	tongue back
3	l-twister	normal: 55 fast: 55	Aa**l**e	/l/	/aː/, /ə/	tongue tip
			Ho**l**e, O**l**e Mo**l**e	/l/	/oː/, /ə/	
4	p-twister	normal: 85 fast: 85	La**pp**en Ha**pp**en	/p/	/aː/, /ə/	lower lip
			ki**pp**en, Si**pp**en, stri**pp**en	/p/	/ɪ/, /ə/	
			klo**pp**en sto**pp**en Scho**pp**en	/p/	/ɔ/, /ə/	
			Pu**pp**en Schu**pp**en	/p/	/ʊ/, /ə/	
5	t-twister	normal: 70 fast: 70	Ve**tt**er Bre**tt**er schme**tt**erte	/t/	/ɛ/, /ɐ/	tongue tip
			hä**tt**e Anne**tt**e gewe**tt**et gefe**tt**et	/t/	/ɛ/, /ə/	
6	s-twister	normal: 190 fast: 185	Preu**ß**en	/s/	/ɔɪ̯/, /ə/	tongue tip and jaw
			mü**ss**en kü**ss**en	/s/	/ʏ/, /ə/	
			pra**ss**en la**ss**en	/s/	/a/, /ə/	
			schmei**ss**en rei**ß**en	/s/	/aɪ̯, /ə/	
			Po**ss**en	/s/	/ɔ/, /ə/	
			fre**ss**en, e**ss**en	/s/	/ɛ/, /ə/	
			Bi**ss**en	/s/	/ɪ/, /ə/	
			Ru**ss**en	/s/	/ʊ/, /ə/	

Note the discrepancy between analyzed items at the fast and normal rates for the s-twisters; for technical reasons, five items had to be excluded from the analysis. Based on the hypotheses we formulated earlier in the paper, we expect differences in the overall speed of these tongue twisters as measured in syllables per second:

According to hypothesis 1, tongue twisters involving a jaw gesture are assumed to be produced much more slowly than tongue twisters containing sound combinations that do not require jaw involvement. The reason is that the mass of the jaw has a slowing effect on the speed of the articulation. In canonical productions of /s/ and /t/ the jaw is involved. However, our speaker realized the /t/ as a flap in which the tongue tip is the sole articulator. Therefore, we predict that the tongue twister containing the flap [ɾ] (as a variant of /t/) will be faster than the s-twister.

According to hypothesis 2, we predict relatively slow speech rates for the k-twister due to the biomechanical constraints at work. Note that we have investigated the VC transition out of a lexically stressed vowel into the following consonant, except for in the case of 'Kakao', where we analyzed the transition of an unstressed vowel into the consonant. Although the stress of a vowel usually has an effect on the articulatory movements, we did not treat these cases separately as there was no crucial difference (with regard to the measurements we made) between the stressed and the unstressed conditions; thus, this choice increased the number of items for our analysis.

Hypothesis 3 argues that tongue twisters involving just tongue tip or lip movement will be very fast. Therefore, we predict that the l-twister, containing many iterations of the lateral liquid /l/, and the p-twister, containing many bilabial stop gestures, can be produced at extremely high rates.

According to hypothesis 4, motor control strategies used in the production of obstruents have an impact on the speed at which they are produced. Fricatives, particularly sibilants, require a finely tuned articulation as a constriction must be formed and the air flow must be funneled towards an obstacle to cause noise with a high intensity. Therefore, stops can be produced faster than fricatives, which implies that overall, the s-twister should be slower than the p-, t-, and k-twisters.

Our fifth hypothesis says that the tC-twister (which is a famous German tongue twister that has been passed down from generation to generation) should be slowest, as it contains many consonant clusters and affricates, which in general involve much greater articulatory effort and tighter coordination than singletons. With our hypotheses, we have estimated the impact of factors that should hamper the overall rate of speech. These factors are the involvement of the jaw, biomechanical characteristics for the production of /k/, the fine motor control necessary in the production of fricatives, and the added complexity in the production of consonant clusters. Overall then, we predict that the t-, l- and p-twisters should be realized with the fastest speech rate, followed by the k-, then the s- and then the tC-twisters.

2.3 Acoustic analysis

As Pfitzinger (2001) points out, a great deal of discrepancy and inconsistency in the investigation, description and definition of speech rate can be found in the literature. To get an evaluation of Georg Winter's overall speech rate, we used the *articulation rate,* as it is described in Laver (1994). The term *articulation rate* may be somewhat misleading, since it implies an articulatory measure while it is actually based on the acoustics. It is frequently referred to in the literature (Künzel, 1987; Laver, 1994) and counts the number of syllables per second (without silent pauses). Künzel (1987) has found that a normal speech rate is characterized by an average of 4.5–5 syllables per second. This value can vary to about 3.5 syllables at slower rates and 7.5 syllables per second at faster rates.

We calculated the articulation rate for each tongue twister at normal and fast speech rates. The duration of each repetition (minus intervening pauses and silences) was divided by the number of actually realized syllables. This includes reduced syllables where a syllable final sonorant retains the syllabicity such as in /lapm/ *Lappen* 'rag' or /ʁʊsn/ *Russen* 'Russians'. After that, an average rate of articulation was calculated for each of the 6 tongue twisters in both rate conditions over the 5 repetitions. We also examined the realization or elision of unstressed schwa in the various iterations of the tongue twisters as detected on the basis of the acoustic envelope and changes in formant structure.

2.4 Articulatory analysis

Opening and closing gestures were analyzed for each individual sound sequence of interest. In order to provide evidence for the properties of the articulators and their control in different segments, the following kinematic parameters were analyzed: the duration of the closing and opening gestures, the actual movement amplitude of these gestures (i.e. the actual distance an articulator travels from one target to the next), and the corresponding velocity peaks of the tangential velocity signal (taking into account the horizontal and vertical components of a movement).

Opening and closing gestures were labeled on the basis of the extrema occurring in the tangential velocity signal. For the closing gesture (see Figure 2), the on- and offsets were defined as extrema from the vowel to the consonant.

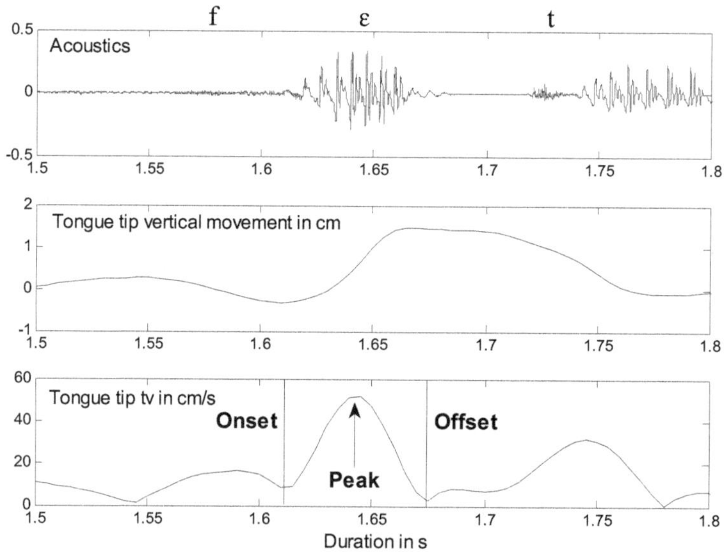

Figure 2: Example of a labeling display for a tongue tip closing gesture for /t/ at a normal rate of speech (acoustic waveform, vertical tongue tip movement, tongue tip tangential velocity).

For the opening gesture on- and offsets were defined as the extrema from the consonant to the following vowel. For two reasons we will focus on the closing gestures in our articulatory analyses: first, the closing gestures in our speech material belong in most cases to the transition between a stressed vowel and an ambisyllabic consonant (first vowel in "Vetter" *cousin* [fɛɾɐ] whereas the following opening gesture refers to a transition from this ambisyllabic consonant toward an unstressed vocalic segment. Hence, there are different conditions in these gestures with regard to the stress on the vowel.
Second, Gracco (1988) points out that the correlation between movement amplitude and velocity is less strong in opening than in closing gestures: in closing gestures, the articulator and muscles involved in forming the consonantal closure are active while in opening gestures, the articulator and muscles involved in the vocalic gesture are active. In our speech material closing and opening gestures often correspond to different articulators and would make a comparison between these gestures difficult.
For the various tongue twisters, different EMA coils were chosen for the analyses: for the tC-, t-, and l-twisters we selected the tongue tip coil, for the s-twister we chose the tongue tip and the jaw coil, for the p-twister the lower lip coil, and for the k-twister the tongue back coil. Lip and tongue movements are not decomposed with regard to the differential jaw contribution, since realistic decomposition is not a straightforward process (Westbury et al., 2002). Note also that we focused more on our speaker's fast speech than on the control condition since he has trained himself to speak fast.

2.5 Statistical analysis

Statistical analyses were carried out using R (Development Core Team, 2008). The articulatory data was submitted to a linear regression analysis. The details of the analysis are given in the relevant results section. In addition, t-tests were calculated to compare the articulation rate of the normal condition with that of the fast condition.

3 Results

In the following sections acoustic and articulatory results for the different tongue twisters are presented.

3.1 Acoustic results

As a first step, all acoustic signals were inspected in order to verify whether Georg Winter's fast speech rate could be attributed to any substantial reduction or deletion of phonemes, syllables, morphemes or even words that go beyond the usual. If listeners were unfamiliar with the tongue twisters and heard Mr. Winter's speech for the first time, his fast tongue twisters were incomprehensible to them. However, since we listened to the acoustic stimuli several times and were familiar with the twisters, we were able to follow his ultra-fast speech. We counted all instances in Georg Winter's speech where there were no traces of an unstressed schwa in the suffix *–en* and assimilation of the following nasal in the spectrogram. The frequency of these occurrences is shown in Table 2.

Table 2. Number of schwa elisions in fast versus normal speech. Note that schwas do not occur very in the t- and k-twisters, therefore they are not included.

Tongue twister	Words with reduced syllables	Speech rate	Amount of schwa elisions
tC-twister	Postkutschkast[ə]n	Normal	10 / 10 (100%)
		Fast	10 / 10 (100%)
l-twister	zwisch[ə]n	Normal	4 / 5 (80%)
		Fast	4 / 5 (80%)
p-twister	Lapp[ə]nschupp[ə]n	Normal	27 / 80 (34%)
	hübsch[ə]n, kipp[ə]n	Fast	80 / 80 (100%)
	stopp[ə]n, stripp[ə]n		
	Robb[ə]nhapp[ə]n		
s-twister	Preus[ə]n, Russ[ə]n	Normal	71 /190 (37%)
	müss[ə]n, prass[ə]n ...	Fast	190/ 190 (100%)

Another interesting finding was the change in the realization of the onset cluster /ʃt/ in the verbs <strippen> and <stoppen> in the p-twister. Georg Winter produced them in different ways in the two speech conditions. In all renditions at the normal rate, [ʃt] was used, concordant with the German standard pronunciation. During the fast rate however, our subject produced a [st] sequence for this cluster, a feature of the Low German dialect of which Georg Winter is a native speaker. It appears that at faster rates, dialectal characteristics are more prevalent in his speech.

These results provide support that Georg Winter's fast speech does not show any extraordinary reductions or deletions which could explain his extraordinarily fast speech rates. In fact, all the information that is necessary for recovering the message is retained in the signal.

As a second step, the articulation rate was calculated for each tongue twister in the two speech conditions. Figure 3 shows that the differences between fast and normal speech conditions are rather large. Tongue twisters differ only marginally at the normal speech rate whereas differences between the different twisters are substantial in the fast rate condition. Articulation rates of over 10 syll/s were found in the t-twister. As predicted, this tongue twister reached the fastest speech rate. Note that the smaller the bar, the lower the rate of articulation, indicating the mean speed for each of the different tongue twister types.

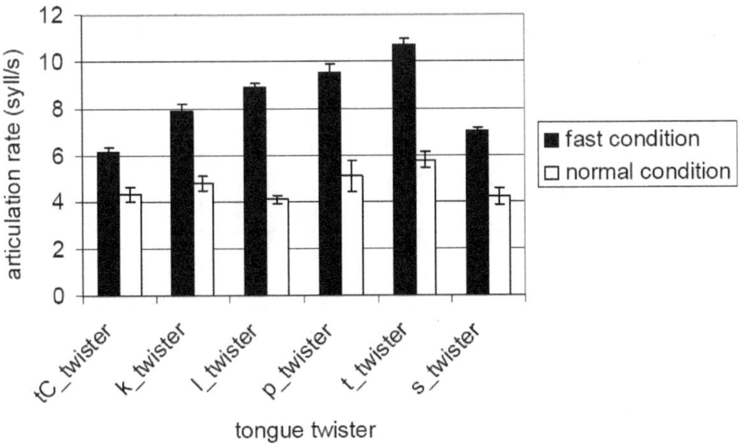

Figure 3: Bar plot with mean articulation rates (syll/s) and standard deviations of the 6 tongue twisters in both rate conditions.

The mean articulation rate calculated over all tongue twisters in the normal speech rate condition was 4.72 syll/s (std.dev. = 0.64) and in the fast speech rate condition 8.39 syll/s (std.dev. = 1.68). Two sided t-tests were conducted to compare the two speech conditions for each tongue twister. All comparisons revealed significant results on a $p<0.02$ level. (We used two-sided t-tests as they are more conservative and because our level of significance was already below $p<0.02$.) An overview of the different average articulation rates that Georg Winter achieved is given in Table 3.

Table 3. Different speech rate measures obtained from the normal and fast productions of the six tongue twisters listed in the appendix. All measures are averaged over the conducted repetitions. Abbreviations: S = mean utterance duration in seconds; Syll = mean number of realized syllables; AR = mean articulation rate; p-value = level of significant difference between the articulation rates in the normal and fast conditions (paired t-test).

No.	Tongue twister	Rate	S	Syll	AR	p-value
1	tC-twister	Normal	7.33	32	4.31	
		Fast	5.22	32	6.13	p<0.001
2	k-twister	Normal	11.97	57	4.78	
		Fast	7.14	56.2	7.88	p<0.001
3	l-twister	Normal	12.2	50	4.12	
		Fast	5.61	50	8.91	p<0.001
4	p-twister	Normal	12.71	64	5.1	
		Fast	6.72	63.8	9.50	p=0.02
5	t-twister	Normal	10.21	59	5.79	
		Fast	5.51	59	10.71	p<0.001
6	s-twister	Normal	17.64	74.6	4.25	
		Fast	10.88	76.4	7.02	p=0.02

Note also that the articulation rate in the normal rate condition is between 4 and 5.5 syllables per second, just as in Künzel's (1987) data. Extreme differences in the two speech rates were found in the t-twister and in the l-twister, where the articulation rate in the faster condition is twice as high as in the normal condition. It seems that these twisters have the most potential to reach extreme speech rates. Note that while the numbers of syllables may be identical in *Kakadu* and *Postkutscher* (both have three syllables), the internal structure of the syllable based on the segmental composition is rather different. *Kakadu* [ka.ka.du] (English: cockatoo) is composed of six sounds, *Postkutscher* [pɔst.kʊtʃ.ɐ] (English: carriage driver) has 8 sounds (the affricate [tʃ] is counted as one sound and may even be ambisyllabic from an articulatory and phonological point of view). In this case a more appropriate measure might have been the phoneme (sound) rate. However, we did not do this comparison because it is only relevant for the complex cluster twister and it would have exceeded the space available to us for this paper.

3.2 Articulatory results

3.2.1 Tangential velocities of the closing gesture

One might expect that our ultra-fast speaker would show differences in peak tangential velocity between the normal and fast conditions. However, as is shown in Figure 4 (upper panel), peak velocities are often similar in the two conditions. T-tests revealed that these peak velocities were not significantly different for the t-, tC-, and l-twisters, which are produced with the tongue tip, whereas significantly lower peak velocities (all with $p<0.001$) were found in the fast speech rate condition for the s-, k-, and p-twisters.

Moreover, in this condition, peak velocities were influenced by sound category, with the fastest rates for /l/, intermediate rates for /p/, /t/, /tC/, a slow rate for /k/ and the slowest rate for /s/. For /s/ we considered the data for the jaw coil, since the jaw is assumed to contribute substantially to the production of the sound. These results are in partial agreement with the acoustic results on the articulation rate, except for the l- and the tC-twisters. In the l-twister, the articulation rate was less extreme than the values measured for peak velocity. Thus, Georg Winter produced the l-twister with an extreme articulatory speed (above 60 cm/s) and an extraordinarily large movement amplitude (up to 4–5 cm); however in terms of the rate of articulation, the l-twister only came in third.

Our speaker shows peak velocity and amplitude values that are up to two or three times faster and larger than commonly reported in the literature for fast speech production (among others Hertrich and Ackermann, 2000; Forrest et al., 1989; Ostry and Munhall, 1985; Jäncke et al., 1995, note that our results are reported in cm/s not mm/s).

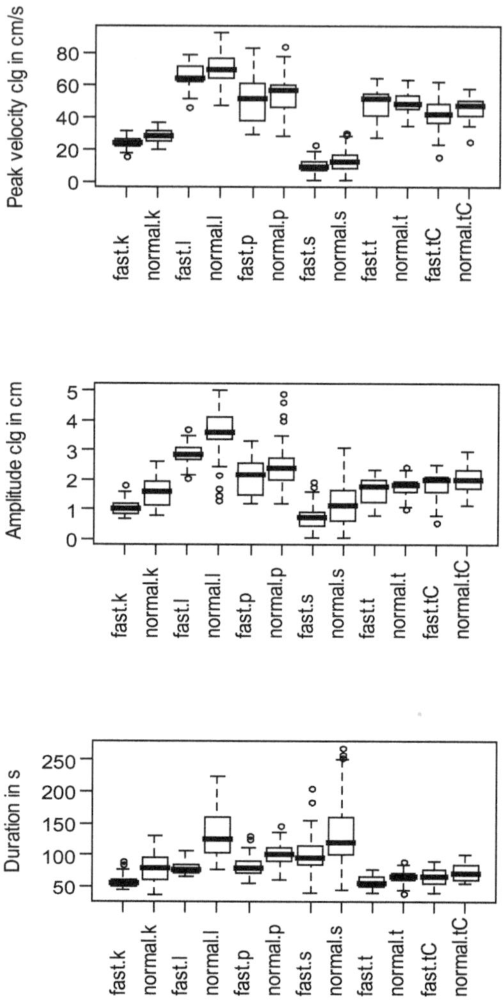

Figure 4: Boxplots showing peak tangential velocity for the respective articulator (note that for /s/, jaw velocity was considered, not tongue tip velocity) in the upper panel, movement amplitude in the middle panel, and duration in the lower panel, for the closing gesture (clg), split by speech rate (fast or normal) and phoneme /k, l, p, s, t, tC/. The boxes range from the 0.25 lower quartile to the 0.75 upper quartile and the inter-quartile distance (size of the box) is henceforth 0.5. The whiskers extend to the 10th and 90th percentiles.

For the tC-twister, the findings on peak velocity may be somewhat misleading, since we only report results from the closing gesture of the first alveolar stop to make it consistent with the other tongue twisters. However, this is only a part of the whole sequence (we are not considering the friction phase or the consonant occurring after that). Differences between t- and p-twisters can also be seen in the acoustics (fast rate), but they are less obvious in the peak tangential velocity data. These variations may result from the fact that for the articulatory measures only closing gestures are considered (VOT reduction may also be crucial, but as mentioned before, this is not of interest to us within the scope of this study), or that schwa-elision occurred more frequently (see Table 2) in the p-twister than in the t-twister. For all other tongue twisters the results of the acoustic and articulatory domain in the fast rate condition match rather well.

To investigate whether the articulatory velocity is dependent on the articulator involved in the production of a particular sound, we fitted two linear models to our data with *peak velocity* as the dependent variable and *articulator* (jaw, tongue tip, tongue back, lower lip) or *sound* (p, t, s, l, tC, or k) as the independent factor. Results for the first model explained 80 % of the variance in the data ($R^2 = 0.80$, df = 922, F = 1239). The model with *sound* as independent factor was slightly better ($R^2 = 0.875$, df = 920, F = 1297), showing that *sound* was a slightly better predictor than *articulator*.

3.3 Movement duration and amplitude

Similar peak velocities in normal and fast speech can only be reached when the movement amplitude of a given gesture is reduced in the fast speech condition. With reduced movement amplitude and similar peak velocity, the overall duration of a gesture will become shorter. Significantly shorter movement durations (see Figure 4, lower panel) were found for all tongue twisters at the fast speech rate in comparison to at the normal rate (at a $p \leq 0.05$ level, except for the tC-twister, where the significance threshold corresponds to about 7 ms, which is close to the temporal resolution of the EMA data). Also, smaller movement amplitudes were found at the fast rate for our speaker (see Figure 4, middle panel): Welch t-tests (taking unequal variance into account) revealed that amplitudes were significantly larger for normal than for fast speech for all tongue twisters, except for /t/. The t-twister did not show significant amplitude reduction; however, on the $p < 0.05$ level, there was a trend in this direction ($p = 0.06$, n.s.), while the tC- and l-twisters reached significance ($p = 0.047$). Amplitude reduction was more substantial in the s-, k-, and p-twisters. Thus, Georg Winter increased speech rate differently with respect to the different articulators. For lower lip, jaw and tongue back movements movement amplitude and tangential velocity were reduced to speed up. For tongue tip movements, while there was no significant difference in the closing gestures in the tangential velocities, movement amplitude was marginally significant.

3.4 On the relation between peak velocity and movement amplitude

The literature is full of experimental evidence that there is a strong linear relation between movement amplitude and velocity even with varying degrees of stress or speech rate (e.g. Kuehn and Moll, 1976; Kelso et al., 1985; Gracco, 1988; Hertrich and Ackermann, 2000; Goozée et al., 2005). This relationship has often been discussed in the light of motor control strategies.

To our knowledge, most of the analyses have focused on bilabial or alveolar stops. In Figure 5 we present our data on different sounds and articulators and in Table 4 we give the corresponding regression analyses. Similarly to previous findings it can be seen that movement amplitude

Table 4. Regression analyses for closing gestures with movement amplitude in dependency on velocity peak, split by phoneme.

Sound	df	Adjusted R2	F	p-value	Articulator
t	128	0.81	551.7	p<0.001	Tongue tip
p	137	0.73	371.7	p<0.001	Lower lip
s	353	0.72	908.4	p<0.001	Jaw
s	353	0.58	495.5	p<0.001	Tongue tip
tC	98	0.56	127.5	p<0.001	Tongue tip
k	88	0.19	22.52	p<0.001	Tongue back
l	108	0.16	21.19	p<0.001	Tongue tip

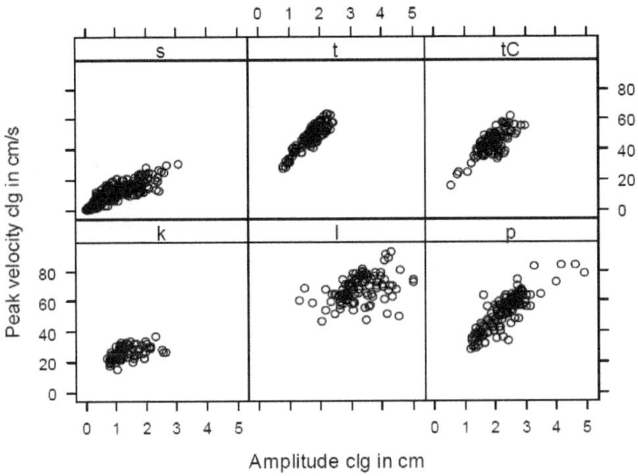

Figure 5: Scatterplots showing peak velocity of the closing gestures (clg, on the y-axis) and movement amplitude (x-axis) for the different sounds. For /s/: jaw velocity; for /t, tC, l/: tongue tip velocity; for /k/: tongue back velocity; for /p/: lower lip velocity.

and peak velocity are tightly linked for all sounds with two exceptions: the l- and the k-twisters. Especially for the l-twister, as the cloud pattern in the graph indicates, large variation was found. In all other cases between 56 % and 81 % of the variance in the data can be explained by means of the linear relation between amplitude and velocity of the respective articulator. Although there is generally a strong link between the two kinematic parameters, the speech sounds differ with respect to the slope of the regression. For the s- (jaw) and k- (tongue back) twisters, a rather low slope is displayed whereas a steeper slope is found for the t-, p-, and tC-twisters. Thus, the relation between movement amplitude and peak velocity may be highly dependent on the articulator involved and/or the realized sound.

4 Summary and discussion

To summarize our main findings: Georg Winter is the fastest speaker of German in Germany (if not in the world) of whom we are currently aware and who has been reported. He is able to realize some tongue twisters with more than 10 syllables per second without any extraordinary acoustic reductions to the point of complete deletions. The acoustic results in the fast speech condition show that the number of syllables he is able to produce per second is highly dependent on the consonants occurring in the tongue twisters: tC < s < k < l < p < t (realized as [ɾ]) in increasing order. Thus, the tC-twister is the slowest (hypothesis 5) and the l-, p-, and t-twisters are the fastest (hypothesis 3; see the modification of this hypothesis in 4). These results are in partial agreement with the articulatory results on the respective peak tangential velocity. In agreement with hypotheses 1 and 2, the s- and the k-twisters were produced with a relatively slow tangential velocity, and the s-twister was produced even more slowly than the k-twister. The t-, p-, and tC-twisters were realized at an intermediate rate, and the l-twisters with an unbeatable maximum of more than 60 cm/s.

Georg Winter produced the tongue tip twisters with similar tangential peak velocities, no matter whether he realized them at the normal or fast speech rate. However, the faster the speech rate, the smaller the movement amplitudes of the tongue tip in these cases. For all other tongue twisters, produced with the jaw, the tongue back and the lower lip, our subject decreased both peak tangential velocity and movement amplitude to reduce the duration of the movement gesture. We also found evidence for the often reported linear relationship between movement amplitude and tangential peak velocity of the closing gesture (with the exception of the l- and k-twisters). The slope of this linear relation differs among the articulators and sounds.

The question arises as to whether the differences in slope could be attributed to the various vowel contexts, which were not controlled for in the different tongue twisters. One can expect that the closer the preceding vowel in articulatory distance (e.g. the distance between /a/ and /s/ in *prassen* is larger than the distance between /ɪ/ and /s/ in *Bissen*), the smaller the movement amplitude, the slower the peak velocity, and the shorter the duration. In order to account for these potential influences, we selected all the tongue twisters where a movement amplitude between 1 and 2 cm was produced and ran another regression analysis (the l-twister had to be excluded since in most cases the amplitudes were larger than that). The slope values of the linear regression were as follows: p-twister: 19.7 (lower lip), t-twister: 19.2 (tongue tip), tC-twister: 16.4 (tongue tip), s-twister: 5.7 (jaw) and 8.4 (tongue tip). For the k-twister there was no linear relation and the velocity was relatively constant. Thus, even when the movement amplitude between the vowel and the consonant was similar, the articulators (jaw versus tongue tip) and the sounds (/s/ vs. /t, p, tC/) differed. Again, results for the tC-twister may be too simple as we only included the first closing gesture for the sake of space.

One last point to note is that we did compare the individual tongue twisters at fast and normal rates with each other, thus, they are perfectly matched for number and occurrence of the target sounds. Moreover, the analyzed sounds are in identical prosodic and segmental positions. When we assessed a ranking between the tongue twisters within the same speech rate, the prosodic position (accentuation status of the word containing the target phone) could not be matched. While we do know (Fougeron and Keating, 1997) that accentuation has an effect on the articulation, for fast and ultra-fast speech our data strongly seem to suggest that this effect is minimized in this rate condition. Even though our speaker made a great effort to rhetorically perform the tongue twisters in the normal rate condition, his realizations at the fast rate were merely the reiteration of acoustic strings without special emphasis on accentuation.

In some instances, we had to rely on phones occurring in words that were prosodically salient, carrying an accent, whereas in another tongue twister, the target phones measured were predominantly located in unaccented syllables. We are not certain as to how strongly this may affect our results.

5 Conclusion

It has been shown that the experimental data support most of our hypotheses presented at the beginning of the paper. Physiological factors and the control mechanisms involved in the production of certain sounds influence the maximal speech rate of the tongue twister. However, it is difficult to tease these factors apart.

We did not expect the l-twister to be as extraordinary as it turned out to be in terms of movement velocity and amplitude. With the exception of clicks (Scharf et al., 1995), tangential velocity values of 70cm/s and movement amplitudes above 4 cm have not been reported in the literature. We attribute the large tongue tip movement amplitude to very low jaw position in this tongue twister. As a consequence, the tongue tip has to move over a long distance from the low vowel to the /l/, developing extreme velocities. In addition, not only a vertical upward movement was observed, but also a horizontal backward movement, similar to a retroflex. These extremely large amplitudes, however, affect the overall movement duration as the l-twister was not the shortest in duration. So far it is unclear why the l-twister did not show a strong relation between movement amplitude and peak tangential velocity. We speculate that either this trade-off does not hold true for all sounds (mostly stops have been analyzed so far) or that the scatter is so large because the tongue tip moves independently in a few repetitions and is more coupled to the rest of the tongue in others.

Apart from the l-twister the question arises as to which strategy Georg Winter used for speaking so fast and precisely without producing speech errors. One of the explanations is certainly the amount of practice he has done and the various exercises he has developed over the years. Such practice has trained his articulatory muscles, fine-tuned coordination between them, and also reduced the amount of planning needed to produce the tongue twisters (it would be very challenging to record brain activity in our subject). Obviously planning would take much longer for spontaneous speech than for highly practiced material. That is, we believe that Georg Winter has trained motor patterns which he can execute at extreme velocities. Moreover, we believe that due to Georg Winter's large movement amplitudes, he did not realize many reductions, deletions or speech errors, despite the extremely high speech rate. In our own experiments with other subjects we have often seen that speakers drastically reduce their jaw oscillations and hold the jaw in a relatively high position to speed up (Fuchs et al., 2009). Such behavior can lead to a complete reorganization of the articulatory coordination (Rochet-Capellan and Schwartz, 2007; Kelso, 1995, for a more general point of view). However, Georg Winter always realized substantial jaw movement. There is hardly any movement amplitude below 0.5 cm (except for a few cases of /s/ in high vowel contexts).

6 Appendix

1. tC-twister
Der Potsdamer Postkutscher putzt
den Potsdamer Postkutschkasten,
der Cottbusser Postkutscher putzt
den Cottbusser Postkutschkasten.

2. k-twister
Warum heißt der Kakao Kakao
und der Kakadu Kakadu?
Wenn der Kakadu Kakao
und der Kakao Kakadu
und der Kaukasus Kakalatsche
und die Latsche Bratsche hieße,
glaubst Du,
dass sich jemand daran stieße?

3. l-twister
Hole Aale, alter Ole,
hole Aale von der Mole,
wo die Aale wohl im Öle
zwischen Pfählen
wählen ihre Höhle,
dort hol deine Aale, Ole,
hole Aale mit dem Zinktopf!

4. p-twister
Bei dem alten Lappenschuppen,
wo die Lappen Schoppen kippen
und für ein paar Robbenhappen
hübsche Lappenpuppen strippen,
bis sich ganze Lappensippen
mit den Rippen von den Robben
um die hübschen Puppen kloppen,
sollst du nie den Schlitten stoppen.

5. t-twister
Als sich der Vetter von Annette
in der Fahrradkette
verheddert hatte
und gewettert hatte,
er wette
jede Wette
dass Annette die Fahrradkette
nicht gefettet hätte,
da schmetterte
der Vetter
auf die Bretter.

6. s-twister
[...]
Preußen müssen Russen,
Russen müssen Preußen prassen
lassen
riesen Bissen essen lassen,
riesen Massen fressen lassen.
Preußen, Russen, Russen Preußen,
essen, fressen, fressen, prassen,
Russen, Preußen, Preußen, Russen
reißen Possen, schmeißen Kissen.
Preußen küssen Russen!
Russen küssen Preußen!

References

Beckman, M., Jung, T., Lee, S., de Jong, K., Krishnamurthy, A., Ahalt, S., Cohen, K., and Collins, M. (1995). Variability in the production of quantal vowels revisited. *The Journal of the Acoustical Society of America*, 97 (1):471–490.

Beckman, M. E. and Edwards, J. (1994). Articulatory Evidence for Differentiating Stress Categories. In Keating, P., editor, *Phonological Structure and Phonetic Form: Papers in Laboratory Phonology III.*, pages 7–33. Cambridge University Press, Cambridge.

Browman, C. and Goldstein, L. (1992). Articulatory phonology: An Overview. *Phonetica*, 49:155–180.

Browman, C. P. and Goldstein, L. (1990). Tiers in Articulatory Phonology, with some Implications for Casual Speech. In Kingston, J. and Beckmann, M., editors, *Papers in Laboratory Phonology I: Between the Grammar and Physics of Speech.*, pages 341–376. Cambridge University Press, Cambridge.

Byrd, D. and Tan, C. (1996). Saying consonant clusters quickly. *Journal of Phonetics*, 24(2):263–282.

Cho, T. and Ladefoged, P. (1999). Variation and universals in VOT: evidence from 18 languages. *Journal of Phonetics*, 27(2):207–229.

Davidson, L. (2006). Schwa elision in fast speech: segmental deletion or gestural overlap? *Phonetica*, 63(2-3):79–112.

Development Core Team, R. (2008). *R: A language and environment for statistical computing. R Foundation for Statistical Computing.*

Forrest, K., Weismer, G., and Turner, G. (1989). Kinematic, acoustic, and perceptual analyses of connected speech produced by Parkinsonian and normal geriatric adults. *The Journal of the Acoustical Society of America*, 85:2608–2622.

Fougeron, C. and Keating, P. (1997). Articulatory strengthening at edges of prosodic domains. *The journal of the acoustical society of America*, 101:3728–3740.

Fuchs, S., Brunner, J., and Busler, A. (2007). Temporal and spatial aspects in the realisations of the voicing contrast in german alveolar and postalveolar fricatives. *Advances in Speech Language Pathology*, 9 (1):34–44.

Fuchs, S., Hartinger, M., Ziervogel, M., and Weirich, M. (2009). *On Coordinative Patterns and Transformation Effects in Reiterant Speech Production.* Poster presented at the Conference Progress in Motor Control, Marseille.

Fuchs, S. and Koenig, L. (2009). The articulation and aerodynamics of voiceless consonants, clusters, and affricates of german. *Journal of the Acoustical Society of America*, 126 (4):1988–2001.

Fuchs, S. and Perrier, P. (2005). On the complex nature of speech kinematics. *ZAS Papers in Linguistics*, 42:137–165.

Fuchs, S., Perrier, P., Geng, C., and Mooshammer, C. (2006). What Role does the Palate play in Speech Motor Control? Insights from Tongue Kinematics for German Alveolar Obstruents. In Harrington, J. and Tabain, M., editors, *Speech Production: Models, Phonetic Processes and Techniques.*, pages 149–164. Psychology Press, New York.

Goozée, J., Stephenson, D., Murdoch, B., Darnell, R., and Lapointe, L. (2005). Lingual kinematic strategies used to increase speech rate: Comparison between younger and older adults. *Clinical linguistics & Phonetics*, 19(4):319–334.

Gracco, V. (1988). Timing factors in the coordination of speech movements. *Journal of Neuroscience*, 8 (12)(12):4628–4639.

Hertrich, I. and Ackermann, H. (2000). Lip–jaw and tongue–jaw coordination during rate-controlled syllable repetitions. *The Journal of the Acoustical Society of America*, 107 (4):2236–2247.

Honda, M., Fujino, A., and Kaburagi, T. (2002). Compensatory responses of articulators to unexpected perturbation of the palate shape. *Journal of Phonetics*, 30(3):281–302.

Jäncke, L., Kaiser, P., Bauer, A., and Kalveram, K. (1995). Upper lip, lower lip, and jaw peak velocity sequence during bilabial closures: No differences between stutterers and nonstutterers. *The Journal of the Acoustical Society of America*, 97:3900–3903.

Jannedy, S. (1995). Fast Speech Reduction in German. In Eckardt, R. and van Geenhoven, V., editors, *CONSOLE II Proceedings*, pages 68–79. Holland Academic Graphics, The Hague.

Kelso, J. (1995). *Dynamic Patterns: The Self-Organization of Brain and Behavior.* The MIT Press, Cambridge, London.

Kelso, J., Vatikiotis-Bateson, E., Saltzman, E., and Kay, B. (1985). A qualitative dynamic analysis of reiterant speech production: Phase portraits, kinematics, and dynamic modeling. *The Journal of the Acoustical Society of America*, 77 (1):266–280.

Kohler, K. J. (1989). Segmental Reduction in Connected Speech in German: Phonological Facts and Phonetic Explanations. In Hardcastle, W. and Marchal, A., editors, *Speech Production and Speech Modelling.*, pages 69–92. Kluwer Academic Publishers, Dordrecht, Boston, London.

Kuehn, D. and Moll, K. (1976). A cineradiographic study of VC and CV articulatory velocities. *Journal of Phonetics*, 4(4):303–320.

Künzel, H. J. (1987). *Sprechererkennung. Grundzüge Forensicher Sprachverarbeitung.* Kriminialistik-Verlag, Heidelberg.

Laver, J. (1994). *Principles of Phonetics.* Cambridge University Press, Cambridge.

Lindblom, B. E. F. (1989). Explaining Phonetic Variation: A Sketch of the H&H Theory. In Hardcastle, W. and Marchal, A., editors, *Speech Production and Speech Modelling.*, pages 403–439. Kluwer Academic Publishers, Dordrecht, Boston, London.

Locke, J. and Pearson, D. (1992). Vocal Learning and the Emergence of Phonological Capacity. A Neurobiological Approach. In Ferguson, C., Menn, L., and Stoel-Gammon, C., editors, *Phonological Development. Models, Research, Implications.*, pages 91–129. Timomium, Maryland.

Löfqvist, A. and Gracco, V. (1997). Lip and Jaw Kinematics in Bilabial Stop Consonant Production. *Journal of Speech, Language and Hearing Research*, 40(4):877–893.

Mooshammer, C., Hoole, P., and Geumann, A. (2007). Jaw and order. *Language and Speech*, 50 (2)(2):145–176.

Munhall, K. and Löfqvist, A. (1992). Gestural aggregation in speech: Laryngeal gestures. *Journal of Phonetics*, 20:111–126.

Ostry, D. and Munhall, K. (1985). Control of rate and duration of speech movements. *Journal of the Acoustical Society of America*, 77:640–648.

Perrier, P., Payan, Y., Zandipour, M., and Perkell, J. (2003). Influences of tongue biomechanics on speech movements during the production of velar stop consonants: A modeling study. *The Journal of the Acoustical Society of America*, 114:1582–1599.

Pfitzinger, H. (2001). Phonetische Analyse der Sprechgeschwindigkeit. *Forschungsberichte (FIPKM)*, 38:117–264.

Rochet-Capellan, A. and Schwartz, J. (2007). An articulatory basis for the labial-to-coronal effect: /pata/ seems a more stable articulatory pattern than /tapa/. *The Journal of the Acoustical Society of America*, 121:3740–3754.

Scharf, G., Hertrich, I., Roux, J., and Dogil, G. (1995). An Articulatory Description of Clicks by Means of Electromagnetic Articulography. In Elenius, K. and Branderud, P., editors, *Proceedings of the 13th ICPhS, Stockholm*, volume 1, pages 378–379.

Takemoto, H. (2001). Morphological analyses of the human tongue musculature for three-dimensional modeling. *Journal of Speech, Language, and Hearing Research*, 44(1):95–107.

Westbury, J., Lindstrom, M., and McClean, M. (2002). Tongues and lips without jaws: A comparison of methods for decoupling speech movements. *Journal of Speech, Language, and Hearing Research*, 45(4):651–662.

Winter, G. (2006). *Zungenbrecher.* Goldmann, Hamburg.

A Note on an Asymmetry in the Hedonic Implicatures of Olfactory and Gustatory Terms

MANFRED KRIFKA

As Samuel Johnson paused to rest on a London park bench one hot summer's day, his profusely sweating bulk caused a young woman sitting next to him to accuse him of smelling. "No, Madam," he replied. "You smell, I stink."

1 The language of the senses

The ways in which languages express primary sense qualities have been investigated quite unevenly, which is due to the fact that there are great differences in how the senses are linguistically represented, which in turn reflects differences in these sense qualities themselves and their role in cognition.

We know most about the sense of Sight, with milestones like Berlin and Kay (1969) and (Kay et al., 2008). Languages differ in quite systematic ways in their expression of color terms that can be related to basic mechanisms of color perception and the further neural processing of visual stimuli. We can distinguish between a pair of terms denoting intensity (*light and dark*), and terms denoting individual colors. There is more to sight than lightness and color, though. Such additional aspects, such as sharp or blurred transitions, have not been investigated by linguists so far.

In contrast, the encoding of the sense of Hearing is little-known territory (but see Dubois, 2000), and would be a rewarding topic for a collaborative project between a phonetician [1] and a lexical semanticist. In English,

1 Already now, I am thankful to Bernd Pompino-Marschall that the occasion of his 60th birthday made it possible that an idea I was pregnant with for about 16 years came to the fore, even if in a still preliminary form. Let's hope that the research project proposed here will not take quite as long to be realized.

there are a number of sound terms: *Loud* and *quiet* or *soft* denote the overall intensity, and thus correspond to *light* and *dark* in the visual domain. We can denote frequency with *high* and *low*, which in other languages may be expressed by the terms for *thin* and *thick* (Shayan et al., 2009). And there are other terms that refer to specific qualities of sound like *clear* or *muffled*. But the typical way in which sounds are expressed in English is by verbs and derived nouns like *bang, whistle, hum* or *whimper.* The terms of Taste have been investigated starting with Myers (1904), with the result that sweet, sour, bitter, salty, *umami* (a Japanese word denoting the taste of monosodium glutamate) and perhaps fatty are frequently distinguished as basic tastes, often with conflations such as common terms for sweet and salty, or sour and bitter (Majid and Levinson, 2008). The sense of Smell is much more diverse, both in the number of sensations it can distinguish and in how they are expressed in languages. While European languages seem to lack genuine descriptive smell terms (Plank and Plank, 1995; Dubois, 2000; Dubois and Catherine, 2002; David, 2002), the Mexican language Totonak is reported to have about twenty, Aschmann (1946). There are no unequivocal terms denoting intensity for Taste or Smell in English; the terms *tasty* or *tasteful* and *tasteless*, or *smelly* come with judgmental connotations, to which I will return below.

For the sense of Touch, English has terms like *rough, smooth, soft* and *hard.* Tactile qualities are often expressed by ideophones in languages that have this word category, cf. Dingemanse (2009). There is no term for denoting general intensity for the sense of Touch. Intensities are again distinguished in terms for the sense of Temperature, as in *hot* and *cold,* with possible terms for temperatures in-between the extremes like *warm* and *tepid.* Pain can also be reported; the general intensity can be expressed by *painful,* and we customarily denote the nature of pain with a few terms, like *stabbing pain.* There are peculiarities with the expression of pain: We find specialized interjections like *ouch,* and there is a close relation to the speech act type of expressives (see Ehlich, 1985; Overlach, 2008, for the expression of pain in language, especially in a clinical context).

The investigation of basic sense terms is beset with problems. One fundamental problem is that it is possible to describe sensory impressions by referring to particular objects – e.g. if the taste of a red wine is called *grainy*, or the smell of a carrion flower is described as *rotten*. In many cases, we would not want to consider such expressions sense terms, but they can develop into true sense terms. For example, the color term *orange* is derived from the common term for *Citrus sinensis*. It can be difficult to decide at which stage the transition to a basic sense term is completed – e.g., what is different, linguistically, between *salty*, a basic taste term related to salt, and *minty*, related to mint? The same problem applies to certain adjectives. If we call a knife *sharp*, does this term primarily refer to the sense quality when we touch it, or is it rather a descriptive term for the property of the knife that happens to create a certain sensation when one touches it?

Another problem is that terms may be semantically restricted, like *blond* for hair (and possibly beer). Terms may encode cross-modal combinations, which is often the case with olfactory and gustatory sense impressions. Also, we find cross-modal terms like *high / low* for pitch, *hot* for taste, or *soft* for reduced loudness. It has been argued by Williams (1976) that such transfers of terms from one sense quality to another follow particular rules, making this area one of the few where regular meaning change can be observed. Viberg (1983) has investigated frequent patterns of non-distinction in the verbs denoting sensory activities; very frequently, for the senses of touch, smell and taste the same verb is used. There is some indication that the linguistic coding of sense impressions is becoming an important research area – witness publications like Plümacher and Holz (2007) and the establishment of a research project on *Language and Perception* at the Max Planck Institute of Psycholinguistics.

2 Pleasantness, with particular reference to smell and taste

In the present article I would like to make a small and rather preliminary contribution to this developing field by pointing out a dimension of perception encoding that is not often talked about, namely the hedonic dimension related to pleasantness (and its opposite, unpleasantness). The dimension of pleasantness is inherently part of nociception, or pain perception. Physical pain is always categorized as unpleasant. This is reflected linguistically by the fact that there are specialized expressive interjections for pain. With the senses of Sight, Hearing, or Temperature, there is no intrinsic relation to pleasantness. It is true that we can react with Ouch! on hearing a balloon pop close to our ears, on touching a hot cooking plate with our hand, or on putting our nose too close to an open bottle of sal ammoniac, but this is because these sensations transcend a threshold where they are classified as painful, and hence unpleasant. With the sense of Smell and Taste there seems to be an intrinsic hedonic bias that is absent with the visual, auditory, tactile or temperature senses (Boisson, 1997; Dubois, 2000, for the sense of smell), and on this I would like to concentrate in this article.

It has been long recognized that the primary dimension for smell words is the distinction between good and bad smells. Buck (1949), in his survey of Indo-European languages, states that

"the only widespread popular distinction is that of pleasant and unpleasant smells [...] and this is linguistically more important than any similar distinction, that is, of good and bad, in the case of other senses."

Boisson (1997) gives evidence for this phenomenon in a number of non-European languages as well; he also observes that the linguistic distinctions for bad smells are generally richer than the ones for good smells. He also states that

"dans toute une série de langues, un terme olfactif neutre (nom ou verbe) employé seul (sans spécification adjectivale or adverbiale) s'interprète comme véhiculant un sens négative,"

and that in language change, a neutral smell word more often develops into a word for bad smells than into a word for good smells. What has escaped notice, though, is that there appears to be the opposite tendency for general words denoting the sense of taste.

The hedonic biases are quite evident with the English terms *tasty* and *smelly*, as the pleasantness and unpleasantness connotations are part of their lexical meanings. The general terms for the olfactory and gustatory are the only terms derived from sense denotations that allow for the formation of adjectives with *–ly*. There is no **seey* or **heary*, and *touchy* has a quite different meaning. And the connotations that they convey are quite contrary, cf. the beginning of the entries of these lemmas in the Oxford English Dictionary:

1. (a) *tasty.* Pleasing to the taste; appetizing, savoury.
   (b) *smelly.* Emitting a bad smell or smells; stinking.

The bias towards pleasantness with the adjective derived from the basic term for taste, and towards unpleasantness with the basic term for smell, is quite remarkable. It is not a quirk of English; inferences about the quality of the English cuisine or the English sanitary standards would be premature. We find the same biases in other languages as well. In German, the verbs for *to smell* and *to taste* can be used intransitively, and they can trigger similar meanings as English *tasty* and *smelly*.

2. (a) *Der Käse schmeckt.* 'The cheese is tasty.'
   (b) *Der Käse riecht.* 'The cheese smells / is smelly.'

English has a similar interpretation of the verb *smell* – see the anecdote about Samuel Johnson at the beginning of this paper. The situation is slightly different from English *tasty* and *smelly*, as pleasantness or unpleasantness is only conveyed by way of cancelable implicature. We can easily modify the intransitive verbs *schmecken* and *riechen* by *gut* or *schlecht*:

3. (a) *Der Käse schmeckt gut / schlecht.* 'The cheese tastes good / bad.'
   (b) *Der Käse riecht gut / schlecht.* 'The cheese smells good / bad.'

The pleasantness implicatures can also be cancelled in other ways. For example, in exclamatives interjections like *mmh!* or *pfui!* can indicate the direction of pleasantness, and corresponding facial expressions can shift the interpretation of the following sentences in either way:

4. (a) *Wie der Käse schmeckt!* 'Oh, how the cheese is tasting!' (good or bad, according to facial expression)
   (b) *Wie der Käse riecht!* 'Oh, how the cheese is smelling!' (good or bad, according to facial expression)

The evidence for the implicatures present in (2) comes from asking German native speakers, but would have to be corroborated by a more serious questionnaire, as well as by corpus studies. Our basic observation is supported by the clear difference in the following sentences; while (a) is strange, as it presupposes that Bernd likes foods that are tasteless or even taste bad, (b) is fine.

5. (a) *Bernd mag den Käse nicht, weil er schmeckt.* 'Bernd doesn't like the cheese because it is tasty.'
   (b) *Bernd mag den Käse nicht, weil er riecht.* 'Bernd does not like the cheese because it is smelly.'

The hedonic implicature appears to be less strong with *riecht*, as the following sentences appear both fine.

6. (a) *Bernd mag den Käse, weil er schmeckt.* 'Bernd likes the cheese because it is tasty.'
   (b) *Bernd mag den Käse, weil er riecht.* 'Bernd does not like the cheese because it has a smell.'

There is interestingly another difference between *schmecken* and *riechen*: While *schmecken* allows for the realization of the experiencer by a dative, this is not possible for *riechen*.[2]

7. (a) *Der Käse schmeckt dem Bernd.* 'The cheese is tasty to Bernd.'
   (b) **Der Käse riecht dem Bernd.*

I do not know, at this point, how this asymmetry in the realization of basic terms for smell and taste generalizes to other languages. It is certainly worth a research project. Here, I would like to speculate about possible reasons for the different behavior of *smell* and *taste*.

3 Explaining the difference between smell and taste

One explanation can be derived from Horn (1984), who discusses the interpretation of *smell*, which comes as a surprise for the theory of autohyponyms developed in his paper. The phenomenon of autohyponyms can be illustrated with such terms like *rectangle* and *square*, where the second is a hyponym of the latter. In this pragmatic configuration, the

2 Realization of the experiencer by dative expressions is not possible for other perception verbs. For pain, interestingly, the experiencer is expressed by the accusative, indicating a greater affectedness: *Der Zahn schmerzt den Bernd.* 'The tooth is hurting Bernd.'

less inclusive term *rectangle* tends to be restricted in its use to those entities for which the more inclusive term cannot be applied. In our case, rectangle will typically be used for rectangles that are not squares. We should expect a similar situation for the terms *smell* and *stink*: The more general term *smell* should be restricted to the complement of those odors that do not fall under *stink*, hence to neutral or good smells. This is not what we find; we rather observe the opposite, a pragmatic strengthening of *smell* to those odors that do not smell so good. Otherwise, Samuel Johnson's remark would not only be not witty; there would have been no grounds for it to begin with, as the lady would have expressed a compliment.

Horn explains this as a politeness effect: Bad smells are often associated with taboos, hence speakers try to avoid talking about them in many situations. They avoid the word *stink* that directly refers to bad smells, and use the originally neutral word *smell* for this case. When this happens regularly, addressees will learn to interpret *smell* in a way that reflects this pragmatic mechanism, as referring to an odor that indeed means bad smells. This implicature has become part of the lexical meaning with *smelly*. If we follow Boisson (1997), this is not a quirk of English, but a wide-spread phenomenon. Boisson also notices that smell terms specific for excrement seem not to exist, which gives further evidence for the role of taboos and euphemisms in this domain.

This explanation sounds plausible, as this is a well-known mechanism for the devaluation of terms via their euphemistic use (Keller, 1994). But the explanation does not work quite as easily for German, which has a term for pleasant smell (*duften*, in addition to *riechen* and *stinken*), yet *riechen* also triggers an implicature of unpleasantness, and *duften* does not broaden its range of application to a general term for olfactory sensation. Horn's explanation is also difficult to apply to the semantic strengthening of *schmecken* towards the meaning of 'tasty'. I am not aware of simple expressions with the meaning 'taste good' or 'taste bad' in English. German has a rather rare verb *munden* for 'taste good', but no simple word for 'taste bad', and so one should prima facie assume that the general term *schmecken* would have a bias towards 'taste bad', contrary to the facts. It is also not possible to invoke euphemisms in this case, as saying that something tastes good is certainly not socially penalized, which would be a precondition for generating a euphemistic strengthening of a neutral term *taste* to a meaning 'taste good'. The second explanation that I would like to offer is based on the assumption that the things that we taste and the things that we smell differ systematically in how pleasant and unpleasant they are. The reason is that we have generally more control over what we put into our mouth than what enters our nose. If one guiding principle of our behavior is the maximization of pleasure, and if there are roughly equally many pleasant and unpleasant smells and tastes available, then we should draw more pleasure out of the sense that we can control, than out of the sense that we cannot control as easily. Consequently, what we taste will be more likely pleasant than what we smell. This is the condition that is known to lead to so-called I-implicatures, the enrichment of meanings to the prototypical case (Levinson, 2000). There are many examples that are structurally similar. For example, *nurse* is typically understood as 'female nurse' because most nurses are female, but this is not part of the lexical meaning – there is no contradiction in *male nurse* (there is even a *Male Nurse Magazine*, see http://www.malenursemagazine.com/). For another example, *'He opened the door.'* is understood to mean that he opened the door in a regular way, but not by smashing the door with an axe, even though we can say *He opened the door with an axe.* I-Implicatures are rooted in the conversational maxim called the I-Principle, which states that speakers should say as little as possible to achieve understanding. The corresponding rule for recipients is to add information that is uncontroversial, conventional and stereotypical.

There is a game-theoretic motivation behind I-Implicatures that can be formulated within bidirectional optimality theory (Blutner, 2000; Jäger, 2002) in a version that factors in the theory of strategic communication (Parikh, 2000). The basic idea is as follows: If we have two expressions α, α' that can express the same meaning m, then the shorter expression is preferred. And if an expression α has two interpretations m, m' then the more likely interpretation is preferred. Let us assume, following the discussion of the different control we exert about taste and smell, that it is more likely that a taste is good than that a taste is bad, and that it is less likely that a smell is good than that a smell is bad. Then we have the following pairs of expressions and interpretations, where ">" expresses preference:

8. *schmeckt*, 'tastes good' > *schmeckt*, 'tastes bad'
   as 'tastes good' is more likely.
   schmeckt, 'tastes good' > *schmeckt gut* 'tastes good'
   as *schmeckt* is less complex.
   schmeckt, 'tastes bad' > *schmeckt schlecht* 'tastes bad'
   as *schmeckt* is less complex.

The overall winner is *schmeckt*,'tastes good': the less complex expression is paired with the most likely interpretation. This blocks the pair *schmeckt gut*, 'tastes good' because it uses a more complex expression. But it does not block the pair *schmeckt schlecht*, 'tastes bad' because in this case we have both a different expression and a different interpretation.
With smelling we have just the opposite configuration if we assume that things that we smell more likely smell bad than good:

9. *riecht*, 'smells bad' > *riecht*, 'smells good',
   as 'smells bad' is more likely.
   riecht, 'smells bad' > *riecht schlecht* 'smells bad'
   as *riecht* is less complex.
   riecht, 'smells good > *riecht gut* 'smells good'
   as *riecht* is less complex.

Here, the pair *riecht*, 'smells bad' comes out as the winner, blocking the pair *riecht*, 'smells good', but the pair *riecht gut*, 'smells good' is not blocked, as it differs in both in form and interpretation from the victorious pair.
In this way we can derive the different pragmatic biases of schmecken 'taste' and riechen 'smell' from general pragmatic rules, together with an apparently well-motivated difference in the likely incidence of good vs. bad smells and tastes.

References

Aschmann, H. (1946). Totonac categories of smell. *Tlalocan*, 2(2):187–189.

Berlin, B. and Kay, P. (1969). *Basic Color Terms. Their Universality and Evolution.* University of Caifornia Press, Berkeley/Los Angeles.

Blutner, R. (2000). Some aspects of optimality in natural language interpretation. *Journal of Semantics*, 17(3):189–216.

Boisson, C. (1997). La dénomination des odeurs: variations et régularités linguistiques. *Intellectica*, 1(24):29–49.

Buck, C. D. (1949). *A Dictionary of Selected Synonyms in the Principal Indo-European Languages. A Contribution to the History of Ideas.* University of Chicago Press, Chicago.

David, S. (2002). *Olfaction, Taste and Cognition.*, chapter Linguistic Expressions for Odors in French., pages 82–99. Cambridge University Press, Cambridge.

Dingemanse, M. (2009). Ideophones and the Senses: The Interplay of Language, Culture, and the Perceptual World in a West-African Society. In *Talk at the workshop The senses in language and culture, 108th AAA Meeting, Philadelphia.*

Dubois, D. (2000). Categories as acts of meaning: The case of categories in olfaction and audition. *Cognitive Science Quarterly*, 1(1):35–68.

Dubois, D. and Catherine, R. (2002). Names and Categories for Odors: The Veridical Label. In Rouby, C., Schaal, B., Dubois, D., Gervais, R., and Holley, A., editors, *Olfaction, Taste and Cognition*, pages 47–66. Cambridge University Press, Cambridge.

Ehlich, K. (1985). The language of pain. *Theoretical Medicine and Bioethics*, 6(2):177–187.

Horn, L. (1984). In defense of privative ambiguity. *Proceedings of the Tenth Annual Meeting of the Berkeley Linguistic Society*, 10:141–156.

Jäger, G. (2002). Some notes on the formal properties of bidirectional Optimality Theory. *Journal of Logic, Language and Information*, 11(4):427–451.

Kay, P., Berlin, B., Maffi, L., and Merrifield, W. (2008). *The World Color Survey.* Stanford: Center for the Study of Language and Information.

Keller, R. (1994). *On Language Change: The Invisible Hand in Language.* Routledge, New York.

Levinson, S. (2000). *Presumptive Meanings: The Theory of Generalized Conversational Implicature.* MIT Press, Cambridge.

Majid, A. and Levinson, S. (2008). Language does provide support for basic tastes. *Behavioral and Brain Sciences*, 31(1):86–87.

Myers, C. (1904). The taste-names of primitive peoples. *British Journal of Psychology*, 1:117–126.

Overlach, F. (2008). *Eine Grammatisch-Semantische und Gesprächsanalytische Untersuchung von Schmerzausdrücken im Deutschen.* Walter de Gruyter, Berlin.

Parikh, P. (2000). Communication, meaning, and interpretation. *Linguistics and Philosophy*, 23(2):185–212.

Plank, F. and Plank, S. (1995). Unsägliche Gerüche: Versuche, trotzdem vom Riechen zu sprechen. In Brandes, U. and Neumann, C., editors, *Das Riechen. Von Nasen, Düften und Gestank*, pages 59–72. Göttingen.

Plümacher, M. and Holz, P., editors (2007). *Speaking of Colors and Odors*. John Benjamins Publishing Co.

Shayan, S., Ozturk, O., and Sicoli, M. (2009). The thickness of pitch: Crossmodal iconicity in three unrelated languages: Farsi, Turkish and Zapotec. *The senses in language and culture Session of the 108th AAA Meeting, Philadelphia*.

Viberg, Å. (1983). The verbs of perception: A typological study. *Linguistics*, 21(1):123–162.

Williams, J. (1976). Synaesthetic adjectives: A possible law of semantic change. *Language*, 52:461–478.

Time for a Shave? Does Facial Hair Interfere with Visual Speech Intelligibility?

SUSANNE FUCHS*
MELANIE WEIRICH
CHRISTIAN KROOS
NATALIE FECHER
DANIEL PAPE
SABINE KOPPETSCH

Abstract: Watching the speaker's face under noisy auditory conditions generally increases the intelligibility of speech. The aim of this study is to investigate the impact of facial hair, covering parts of the articulators, on visual speech intelligibility under noise. We hypothesized that facial hair decreases intelligibility, leads to a longer response time and a lower confidence to perceive the relevant target word. Thus, is it time for a shave now? Three speakers were recorded with a video camera in three different conditions: wearing no beard, a moustache and a long chin beard. Speakers uttered the relevant sentences in all three conditions. These video recordings provided the basis for an audio-visual perception experiment: 44 subjects, in three separate groups, perceived either the speakers in the no beard condition or the moustache condition or the long chin beard condition. Audio only and audiovisual data were presented. Subjects were instructed to type in a text input field what they perceived. Their response time was measured. Our findings show that the impact of facial hair (moustache) on speech intelligibility is generally rather small and not significant, but subjects seeing speakers with a moustache improve more from the audio only to the audiovisual condition in comparison to those who see speakers with no beard. Moreover, they need a longer response time and they are less confident to perceive the relevant target word. We interpret this result with respect to a greater attentiveness when subjects are confronted with visual impoverishment of the articulators.

* Over the last year I tried very hard to get a similar beard to yours, Bernd (just for this experiment). I hope yours will never be totally shaved.

1 Introduction

If one walks through the first level of the main building at the Humboldt University in Berlin and looks at all the portraits of researchers who studied there, became professors, and in some cases won a Nobel prize, one may come to the conclusion that the most important visible sign for a famous person is to be a man and to have a beard. About 80 per cent of the various portraits in this gallery show men with a beard (except for some of the philosophers and the women), independent of the generation. Nowadays, this trend might be in a transition towards a more beardless fashion, since more females become famous and the equipment to shave facial hair has improved. However, in our community of speech researchers, there is clearly no lack of famous men with facial hair (see Figure 1). This paper is not concerned with the social status attributed to facial hair on a man (see Appendix for some recent contributions in magazines on this topic), but with the influence of facial hair on audio-visual speech intelligibility in noise.

It is generally known that watching the speaker's face increases the intelligibility of speech in noisy environments (Sumby and Pollack, 1954; Grant and Seitz, 2000). By observing the cyclical opening and closing of the visible jaw, one may be able to identify the rhythmic structure of the spoken utterance or even the focus of a particular sequence (Dohen et al., 2005). Moreover, certain minimal pairs, e.g. the /m/-/n/ contrast, may be better identified with the additional visual information of their articulators than with only the purely acoustic information (Schwartz et al., 2002). Facial hair can cover parts of the face such as the upper lip, the teeth or the larynx. If the upper lip, teeth and tongue movement are partially hidden due to facial hair, the area of the mouth opening is modified, and facial hair is responsible for a kind of *natural visual impoverishment* of the visual intelligibility of speech. Under normal auditory conditions such an impoverishment may be marginal for the intelligibility of speech, since the auditory information is fully available. However, under noisy auditory conditions, the visual cues may be crucial for increasing speech intelligibility.

Based on these considerations, we hypothesize that:

1. Facial hair hiding visible articulatory movements leads to lower speech intelligibility under noisy auditory conditions, a longer re-

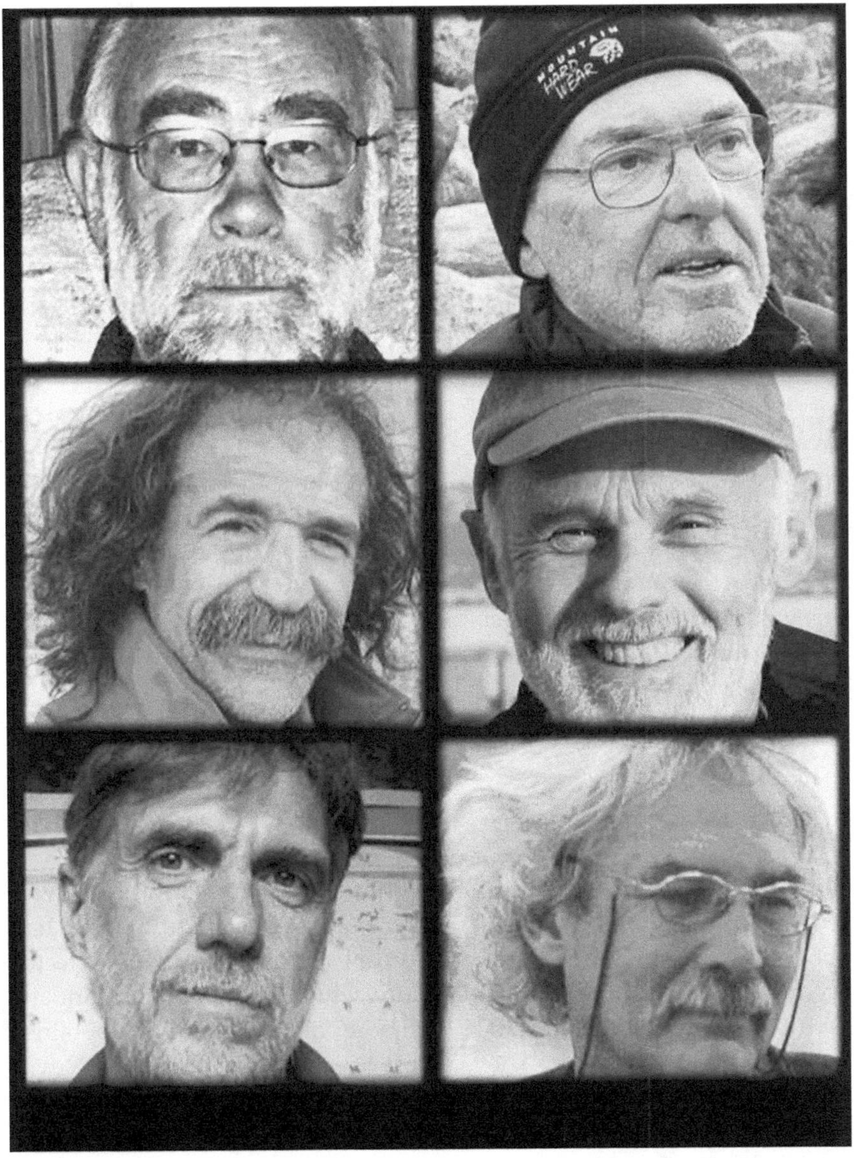

Figure 1. Well-known researchers from the area of speech production and perception with various beard shapes. All photos have been printed with the permission of the individuals.

sponse time, and a lower confidence in recognizing the relevant target words.

2. The shape and location of the beard is crucial for the reduced intelligibility in noise. A moustache hiding the upper lip movement has a larger impact on visual speech intelligibility than a long chin beard, hiding the larynx only.
   So in terms of speech intelligibility is it now time for a shave or not?

2 Methodology

Investigating the interference of facial hair with visual speech intelligibility poses the problem of accurately controlling the amount and shape of facial hair across several speakers while at the same time keeping the recording situation constant. Since it is difficult to find participants willing to grow and then cut their beards as needed for this study and since this would lead to large time spans between the recordings, we decided to use artificial beards made from natural hair. Two different beard types were chosen, a moustache and a long chin beard.

2.1 Stimuli

2.1.1 Video recordings

Three male speakers (hereafter SP1, SP2, and SP3) in their mid 20s were recorded (see Figure 2). None of them had substantial natural facial hair above 3mm during the time of the recording. The speakers were selected according to their hair colour and texture, which had to fit the colour and texture of the attached facial hair. Two types of facial hair were obtained in a specialist mask shop. They consist of natural hair which is woven into a strip of gauze that provides an attachment area. With the help of professional glue (Mastix) used in the film industry, the gauze strip was attached to the facial surface.
Every speaker read a set of 40 sentences (each of the 20 target words in two different carrier sentences) in three conditions: with no beard (beard0), with the moustache (beard1), and with the long chin beard

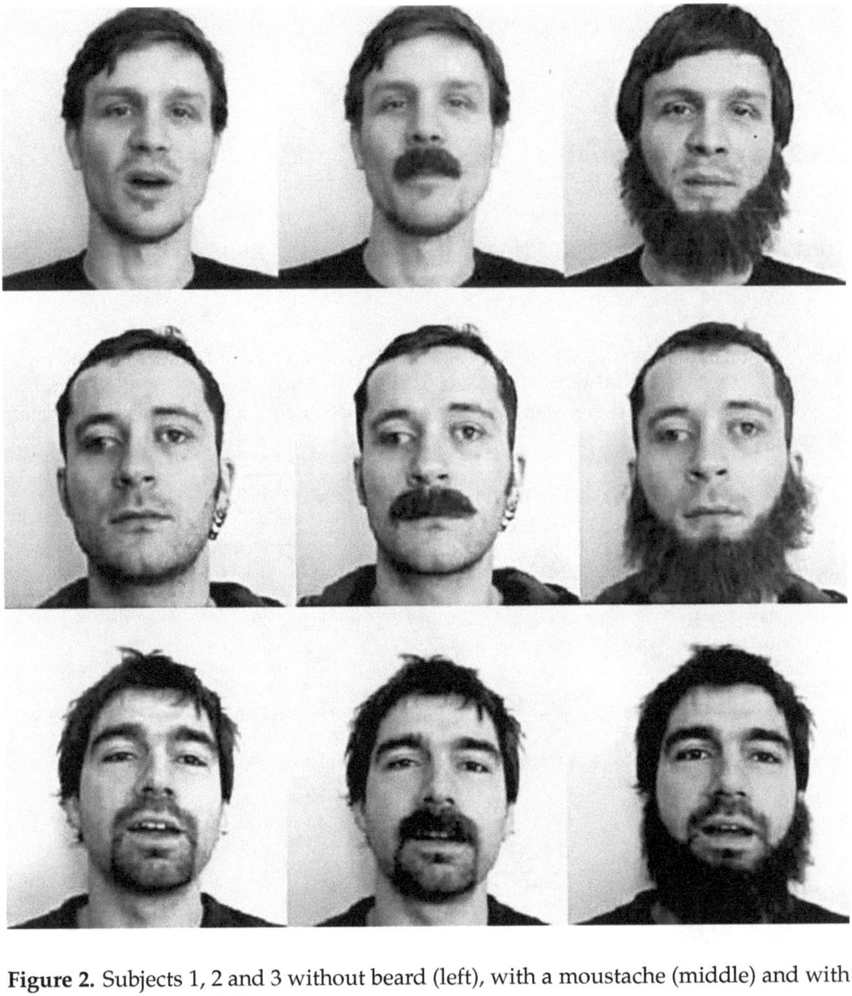

Figure 2. Subjects 1, 2 and 3 without beard (left), with a moustache (middle) and with a long chin beard (right).

(beard2). The recordings were carried out in a soundproof room at the Centre of General Linguistics (ZAS) in Berlin using a Sony DCR-TRV14E video camera. The speaker was seated approximately 80 cm away from the camera in front of a uniformly white background and was uniformly lit. The video frame comprised the entire head and neck of the speaker. The recording time was about 10 minutes per speaker.

2.1.2 Speech material

Twenty nouns were selected as target words on the basis of their high frequency in the lexicon (Haas et al., 1984) and their semantic content (see Table 1).

Table 1. Speech material with target words (English translation), phonological structure and IPA (Standard German), frequency in the lexicon, and number of voiceless obstruents.

TARGET WORD	PHONOLOGICAL STRUCTURE AND IPA	FREQUENCY	NO. OF VL. OBSTRUENTS
Abend (evening)	VCVCC /aːbənt/	129	0
Beispiel (example)	CVVCCVC /baɪʃpiːl/	774	2: /ʃp/
Beruf (job)	CVCVC /bəruːf/	342	1: /f/
Bücher (books)	CVCVC /byːçɐ/	128	1: /ç/
Dinge (things)	CVCV /dɪŋə/	216	0
Freude (happiness)	CCVVCV /frɔɪdə/	158	1: /f/
Kinder (children)	CVCCVC /kɪndɐ/	628	1: /k/
Klasse (class)	CCVCV /klasə/	180	2: /k, s/
Leben (life)	CVCVC /leːbən/	215	0
Leute (people)	CVVCV /lɔɪtə/	544	1: /t/
Mädchen (girl)	CVCCVC /meːdçən/	198	1: /ç/
Musik (music)	CVCVC /muziːk/	156	1: /k/
Schule (school)	CVCV /ʃuːlə/	719	1: /ʃ/
Seite (side)	CVVCV /zaɪtə/	187	1: /t/
Sommer (summer)	CVCVC /zɔmɐ/	249	0
Strasse (street)	CCCVCV /ʃtraːsə/	142	3: /ʃ, t, s/
Vater (father)	CVCVC /faːtɐ/	289	2: /f, t/
Wasser (water)	CVCVC /vasɐ/	163	1: /s/
Wetter (weather)	CVCVC /vɛtɐ/	206	1: /t/
Woche (week)	CVCV /vɔxə/	181	1: /x/

Their meaning had to fit four carrier sentences without allowing the prediction of the target word from the semantic context of the carrier sentence. There were four carrier sentences:
Meine Freundin hat __ gesagt. *(My friend said __.)*
Auf dem Blatt hat __ gestanden. *(__ was written on the paper.)*
Meine Mutter hat __ geschrieben. *(My mother wrote ___ .)*
Mein Nachbar hat __ geschrien. *(My neighbour cried __ .)*
For the video recording every target word occurred in two of the four carrier sentences, but for further analysis only one of the two sentences was selected to make the perception experiment feasible in terms of its duration. Target words are all bi-syllabic. In general, we tried to make the corpus as phonetically balanced as possible (see Table 1).

2.1.3 Stimuli processing

From the continuous video recording short clips of equal length were extracted containing one sentence each. The starting point was set at 0.5s before the speaker uttered the first syllable and the endpoint at 0.5s after the completion of the sentence. Using Adobe Premiere 1.0 the original video frames of 720 x 576 pixels were cut on the left and right side to be square-sized (576 x 576 pixels) and if necessary, slightly adjusted in size to position all speakers at the exact same size at the exact same location in the frame. The original sound track was extracted and its average loudness computed. Commercial multi-speaker babble noise was added with its loudness set to result in a final signal-to-noise ratio of 3dB. For the audio-only condition the video frames showing the speaker were replaced by black frames. The acoustic signals were low-pass filtered at 12dB/octave with a cut-off frequency of 8000 Hz in order to remove high-frequency noise from the recording and, more importantly, to match the frequency range of the stimuli to the frequency range of the multi-speaker babble noise.

2.1.4 Design

To avoid any participant seeing the same speaker with different beards and becoming aware of the aim of the study, the beard condition was made a between-subject factor while 'speaker' was kept within-subject.

Thus, a participant would see all three speakers with the same beard type. Furthermore, despite the fact that each speaker was recorded in all beard conditions in a single session, changes in the acoustics among the different beard conditions cannot be ruled out. The audio-only control condition (A) was designed to mirror the audio-visual (AV) condition: The audio data in the A condition are the same as those in the AV condition, but they are presented with a black video. Each target word plus carrier sentence was presented in six different versions (beard0-AV, beard1-AV, beard2-AV, beard0-A, beard1-A, beard2-A), not counting repetitions.

2.1.5 Procedure

The experiment control software Alvin (see Hillenbrand and Gayvert, 2005) was used to present the stimuli on a monitor and register the participants' responses. The participants were seated approximately 50cm away from the monitor and listened to the stimuli via Sennheiser HD 201 headphones. They were instructed to type the target word into a text input field on the screen using the computer keyboard as soon as they thought they had recognized it after (or while) watching the stimulus video clip. They were told that their response times were measured by pressing the enter button after they typed in the perceived word. Subjects were subsequently prompted to rate their confidence in having correctly identified the target word on a 5-point Likert scale by pressing a software button with the computer mouse. The test trials (20 target words * 6 conditions * 2 repetitions) were preceded by 5 practise trials. The experiment took approximately 30 minutes.

2.1.6 Participants

Forty-six participants took part in the experiment. Two of them had to be excluded after the experiment as it became apparent that they were (for different reasons) familiar with the target words. The participants were randomly assigned to one of three stimuli groups (speakers without beard, speakers with a moustache, speakers with a long chin beard) though across groups the same gender ratio (4 males, 11 females, except beard1 with only 10 females) and a similar age range (between 20 and

35 years) were maintained. The participants received 10 Euro.

2.1.7 Statistical design

The statistical package R (Development Core Team, 2008) was used for further quantitative analyses. Since our dataset was not equally well balanced (only data from 14 subjects were included in the beard1 condition whereas data from 15 speakers were included in the beard0 and beard2 conditions), we used mixed models. Mixed models consist of fixed effects and random effects. Beard condition (beard0, beard1, beard2) served as the fixed effect and listener and target word as random effects. Since the listeners identification of the relevant target word was either correct (1) or false (0) and the data are therefore binomial, mixed models of the family binomial were run. For continuous data like reponse time, a linear mixed model was used and the corresponding pMCMC values were calculated. pMCMC values are similar to the classical p-values but rely on the **M**onte **C**arlo **M**arkov **C**hain method. The details are given in the results section.

3 Results

Intelligibility: There is clear evidence that speech intelligibility increases when watching the speaker's face (AV) in comparison to the audio-only (A) condition. This increase is on average 17 % for no beard, 20 % for the moustache and 12 % for the long chin beard (see Figure 3). Speakers with a moustache have in all cases the lowest speech intelligibility, whereas speakers with a long chin beard have a similar or even better intelligibility in comparison to speakers with no beard. Running a mixed model for the audio only data with beard condition as the fixed factor and listener and target word as random factors provides evidence that beard condition has an effect in the following way: beard0 differs significantly from beard1 ($z=-2.029$, $p=0.0425$), but not from beard2 ($z=1.886$, $p=0.0593$) and beard1 from beard2 ($z= 4.063$, $p<0.001$). In the audiovisual condition beard condition had no impact on intelligibility. This result is surprising, since we expected an effect of beard condition in the audiovisual condition, not in the audio only condition (we will come to an explanation at a later point). *Response times*: Response times were first transformed into a

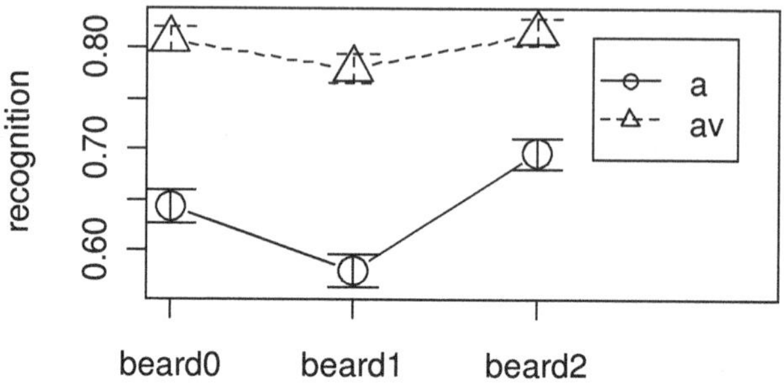

Figure 3. Means and standard errors for target word recognition; a = audio data (circle markers), av = audio-visual data (triangle markers), 3 beard conditions: beard0 = no beard, beard1 = moustache, beard2 = long chin beard.

logarithmic scale to make them more normally distributed. Second, we checked whether the mixed model (in this case we ran a linear mixed model, since the data are continuous) provided a good fit to the data. A quantile-quantile plot showed that the model was stressed when it tried to fit the longest response times. Hence, we removed the extreme outliers with a standardized residual at a distance greater than 2 standard deviations from zero (trimmed model in Baayen (2008, ch.7)). These extreme outliers (up to 22000 ms) were probably due to typos or to the fact that listeners forgot to press the enter button after typing the relevant word.

Our findings provide evidence that response times are similar for the A and AV data (Figure 4); hence we pooled all data together. However, results differ significantly with respect to the beard condition. Subjects showed significantly longer response times in the beard1 condition (moustache) in comparison to beard0 (pMCMC=0.0042) and beard2 (pMCMC=0.0001). *Listeners' confidence*: Similarly to intelligibility, subjects were most confident on a 5-point Likert scale when they rated the AV data for the speakers with a long chin beard (Figure 5). They were least confident when they rated the audio-only data for speakers with a moustache. The confidence level was significantly larger in the audiovideo condition than in the audio-only condition (pMCMC>0.001) for all beard types. Doing pairwise comparions, confidence ratings were

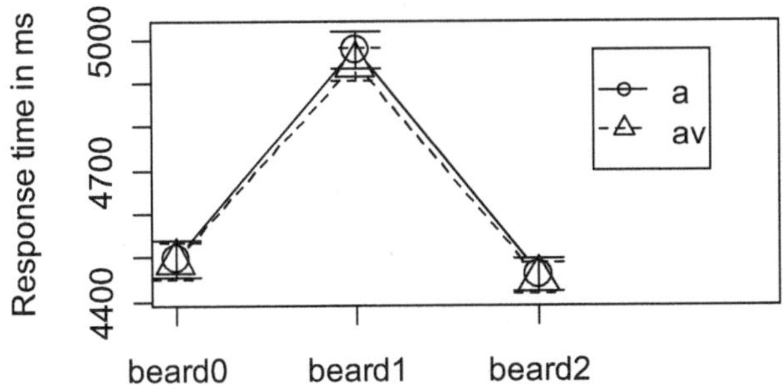

Figure 4. Means and standard errors for response times (real data in ms); a = audio data (circle markers), av = audio-visual data (triangle markers), 3 beard conditions: beard0 = no beard, beard1 = moustache, beard2 = long chin beard.

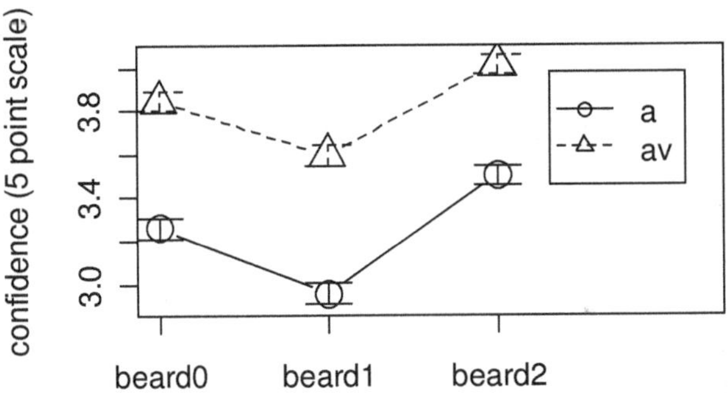

Figure 5. Means and standard errors for confidence ratings; a = audio data (circle markers), av = audio-visual data (triangle markers), 3 beard conditions: beard0 = no beard, beard1 = moustache, beard2 = long chin beard.

significantly different only between beard1 (moustache) and beard2 (long chin beard) in the AV condition (pMCMC=0.0058) and in the A condition (pMCMC=0.01).

So far facial hair had some impact on intelligibility, response time and also confidence. However, dif reduced intelligibility for the moustache in comparison to the no beard condition, the findings for the long chin beard go against our expectations. Speakers wearing a long chin beard were perceived with a greater intelligibility in comparison to the no beard condition in the audio only condition. Moreover, it is surprising

that facial hair in the audio-only condition showed an effect of the beard, although no visual information is available. Two explanations might be possible for this finding: First, since the A and AV conditions were presented randomly and the number of target words was limited to keep the experiment feasible, a strong learning effect could have taken place. Hence, listeners may even become better when they have no visual information available, since they have learnt the relevant target word.
Second, facial hair covering the upper lip (moustache) could have influenced the lip radiation and may have influenced the acoustic signal. Such an explanation seems plausible, since beard2 does not show an effect and it does not cover the lip area.
Third, since we glued the beards on the facial skin of the speakers, it may have caused some irritation, so that our speakers produced the relevant sentences in a different way with the long chin beard in place. During the recording session which lasted only about 10 minutes per speaker and during the data preparation, we were not aware of such an effect, thus we assume a learning effect.

3.1 Learning

To check the potential effects of learning, all the A and AV data were pooled together, but recognition was split by beard condition and occurrence of the target words from the first to the sixth trial (see Figure 6). Figure 6 displays the results and clearly shows an effect of learning.

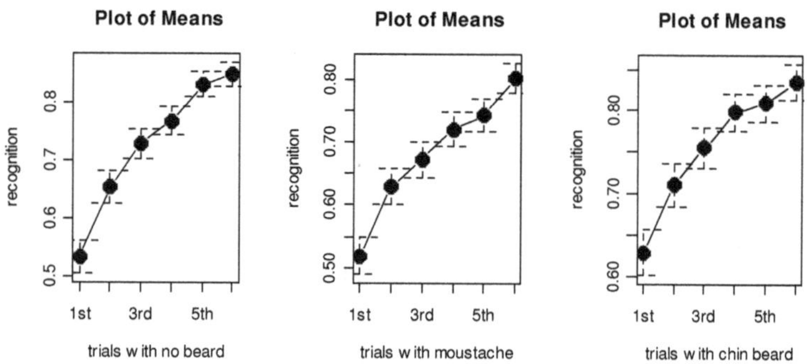

Figure 6. Means and standard errors of recognition rate (A and AV data pooled together) split by beard condition (from left to right) and trial.

The recognition rate increases from one trial to the next, independently of the beard condition. The learning effect is greatest from the first trial of a word to the second one. Next we ran a mixed model for the first trial only to test whether differences between the beard conditions are already evident in the first trial.
No statistical differences were found comparing beard0 with beard1 ($z=-0.4664$, $p=0.6409$) on the first trial. However, beard1 differs marginally from beard2 ($z=1.9614$, $p=0.0498$). This result leads us to conclude that our speakers used different strategies when wearing a long chin beard. We can only speculate about these strategies. One of the reasons might be that for the long chin beard, opening the jaw stretches the surface of the skin, but the artificial beard did not stretch as much as the skin. Such a difference might have caused a different speaking behaviour of our subjects. These results would be in agreement with recent findings on the effects of skin stretching on speech production and perception by Ito and colleagues (Ito et al., 2009). Although this finding could be very interesting for the role of somato-sensory information in speech production and perception, it is disruptive for our perception experiment, since it is difficult to derive any reliable conclusions when comparing the long chin beard with the other conditions. Hence, we will only discuss the comparison between no beard and the moustache.

3.2 Word effects

Splitting intelligibility by the different words used in this corpus reveals a large impact of the individual word. Words like *Leben* (life), and *Woche* (week) have a relatively low recognition rate in the audio-only condition and their intelligibility increases substantially (up to about 40%) in the AV condition. An intermediate improvement was found for words like *Abend*(evening) or *Freude* (happiness). All other words, e.g. *Strasse* (street), *Mädchen* (girl), show a lower difference between the A and the AV conditions and in most cases words are already recognized successfully in the A condition (above 80 percent). These differences among the words cannot be explained with respect to the variation in word frequency presented in Table 1. We noticed that in the word group with a high intelligibility in the audio-only condition, voiceless obstruents occur relatively often. Voiceless obstruents, in particular voiceless fricatives, are perceptually very salient (Balise and Diehl, 1994) and might therefore be recognized even under noisy auditory conditions. At this point, we present the intelligibility plots for the group of 0 obstruents and the group of 2 obstruents (for 3 obstruents the sample size is rather small) in the no beard and moustache conditions.

In Figure 7 it can be seen that the number of voiceless obstruents in bisyllabic words has an impact on the intelligibility in the two selected cases. If the target word includes no voiceless obstruents, the improvement from A to AV is larger in the no beard condition than in the moustache condition and the no beard AV condition is significantly better than the moustache.

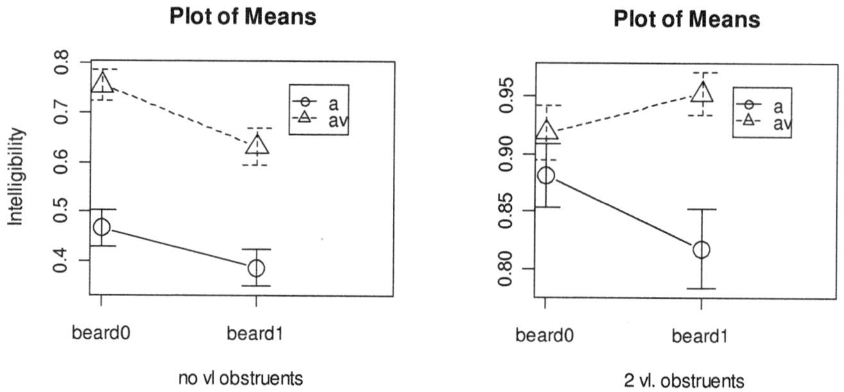

Figure 7. Means and standard errors of intelligibility split by number of obstruents in the target word: left subplot: 0 voiceless obstruents, right subplot: 2 voiceless obstruents, a = audio, av = audiovisual condition, beard0: left column, beard1: right column.

Similar differences are not evident in words with two voiceless obstruents, where intelligibility for no beard is already 90 per cent in the audio-only condition and it is not significantly different from the AV condition. For the moustache (beard1) the results for AV-condition improve in relation to the audio only condition, but within a given condition (A or AV) the findings for no beard and beard1 do not differ.

4 Summary and conclusion

We have good news for all those who have facial hair longer than 3 mm: There is no need to shave! Although a trend towards reduced intelligibility was found in the beard1 condition (moustache), this trend was not significant in the audiovisual condition. Moreover, the improvement from the audio-only to the audio-visual condition is larger for beard1 (moustache) than beard0 (no beard), mainly due to the lower intelligibility of the moustache in the audio only condition. We interpret this result with respect to a learning effect from the first presentation of the target word to later occurrences and a greater attentiveness. Listeners who are presented with an impoverished visual signal have to memorize target words to a greater extent and they pay more attention to this visual information, thereby enhancing intelligibility. The greater attentiveness may also be reflected in the significantly longer response time found for beard1. Thus, if you wear a moustache in a noisy auditory environment, please do not speak fast and take a break from time to time, otherwise listeners may not be able to process your speech. Moreover, be aware that people may be attracted by your beard and focus on it (that may be relevant particularly for politicians). Similar to the findings for intelligibility, listeners show a non significant trend towards greater confidence that they have perceived the right word when they see speakers without any facial hair in comparison to when they see speakers wearing a moustache. However, findings are influenced by the number of voiceless obstruents in a given word: the more voiceless obstruents in a word, the easier the recognition of the word even under auditory noise. We interpret this result with respect to the perceptual salience of these sounds. Based on our data, we were not able to verify whether differences in the shape of the facial hair would affect intelligibility. Such an investigation may be carried out in the future.

5 Appendix

Sächsische Zeitung 27th / 28th of june 2009, front page

"Haare im Gesicht sind Männersache – ob es den Frauen gefällt oder nicht..... Da soll doch einer sagen, Bärte seien nicht gut für die Karriere....Zeige mir was in deinem Gesicht wächst und ich sage dir, wer du bist."

Facial hair is man's business – whether it suits women or not....How can one dare to say facial hair would not be good for the career.... Show me your facial hair and I will tell you who you are.

Page M5:

"Geschichten im Gesicht"
"Bärte sind mehr als nur Haare am Kinn. Sie machen aus Männern Charakterköpfe mit Markenzeichen."

Facial hair is more than only hair on the chin. It makes striking heads out of men.

Prince, September 2009, page 130

"Seitdem Brad Pitt, George Clooney und andere Hollywoordstars nicht mehr oben ohne herumlaufen, hat der Schnäuzer die Straßen zurückerobert. Ist der Hype berechtigt?"

Ever since Brad Pitt, George Clooney and other Hollywood stars do not walk about topless, the moustache is back on the streets. Is the hype justified?

"Im Volksmund wird der Schnäuzer auch "Rotzbremse", "Suppensieb", "Popelfänger", "Schenkelbürste" oder "Pornobalken" genannt. "

In vernacular speech the moustache is also called "snot bracket", "soup filter", "bogey catcher", "crural brush" or "porn baulk".

"Träumt eine Frau von einem Mann mit Schnäuzer, hat das laut Esoterikanbieter Traumdeuter.ch folgende Bedeutung: Ein Mann, den Sie immer für einen Helden hielten, entpuppt sich als armseliger Tropf."

If a woman dreams about a man with a moustache, it has the following meaning according to the esoteric web-site Traumdeuter.ch: A man, who you always took for a hero, turns out to be a poor blighter.

"Schnurrbärte sind eine Bakterienschleuder."

Moustaches are bacteria catapults.

"Salvador Dali war der festen Überzeugung, mit seinen Schnurrbartspitzen göttliche Botschaften empfangen zu können."

Salvador Dali had the firm conviction that he would pick up divine messages through the tips of his moustache.

"Heute brauchen Typen dicke Karren., früher reichte der dickste Schnurrbart: Zu Kaiserzeiten wies die Größe des Soldatenschnäuzers auf den Rang innerhalb der Armee hin."

Nowadays, guys need big cars, in former times the largest moustache was sufficient: In the days of the German Kaiser the size of the soldier's moustache was a sign of status in the army.

"Man kann sich mit seinem Schnurrbart auch in Geduld und Selbstdisziplin üben: Der Inder Badamsinh Juwansinh Gurjar ließ seinen Schnäuzer in 25 Jahren auf knapp vier Meter Länge wachsen – Weltrekord."

One can also exercise patience and self-discipline with a moustache: The Indian Badamsinh Juwansinh Gurjar grew his facial hair for 25 years, reaching a length of almost 4 metres – world record.

6 Acknowledgements

We would like to thank Jörg Dreyer for the technical support, all participants of this study, Sandra Pape-Hagushikowa for the graphical design of Figure 1, all researchers who provided their photos, and Jean-Luc Schwartz for useful comments on an earlier version of this paper. This work was supported by a grant from the BMBF to the PB1 at ZAS. It is dedicated to all men with facial hair and Dieter Fuchs.

References

Baayen, R. (2008). *Analyzing Linguistic Data: A Practical Introduction to Statistics Using R*. Cambridge University Press.

Balise, R. and Diehl, R. (1994). Some distributional facts about fricatives and a perceptual explanation. *Phonetica*, 51(1-3):99–110.

Development Core Team, R. (2008). *R: A language and environment for statistical computing. R Foundation for Statistical Computing.*

Dohen, M., Loevenbruck, H., and Hill, H. (2005). A Multi-Measurement Approach to the Identification of the Audiovisual Facial Correlates of Contrastive Focus in French. *Auditory-visual processing workshop, British Columbia*, pages 115–116.

Grant, K. and Seitz, P. (2000). The use of visible speech cues for improving auditory detection of spoken sentences. *The Journal of the Acoustical Society of America*, 108:1197–1208.

Haas, W., Knetschke, E., and Sperlbaum, M., editors (1984). *Textkorpora 1: Einführungs- und Registerband.* PHONAI, Lautbibliothek der deutschen Sprache 28. Max Niemeyer Verlag, Tübingen.

Hillenbrand, J. and Gayvert, R. (2005). Open source software for experiment design and control. *Journal of Speech, Language, and Hearing Research*, 48(1):45–60.

Ito, T., Tiede, M., and Ostry, D. (2009). Somatosensory function in speech perception. *Proceedings of the National Academy of Sciences USA*, 106(4):1245–1248.

Schwartz, J., Abry, C., Boë, L., and Cathiard, M. (2002). Phonology in a Theory of Perception-for-Action-Control. In Durand, J. and Laks, B., editors, *Oxford Studies in Theoretical Linguistics*, pages 254–280. Oxford University Press, New York.

Sumby, W. and Pollack, I. (1954). Visual contribution to speech intelligibility in noise. *Journal of the Acoustical Society of America*, 26(2):212–215.

Kolibri 360 GmbH
Ferdinand-Jühlke-Straße 7
99095 Erfurt, Deutschland
produktsicherheit@kolibri360.de